Racial and Ethnic Patterns of Mortality in New Mexico

Racial and Ethnic Patterns of Mortality in New Mexico

EDITED BY

Thomas M. Becker
Charles L. Wiggins
Rita S. Elliott
Charles R. Key
Jonathan M. Samet

University of New Mexico Press
ALBUQUERQUE

Copyright © 1993
by the University of New Mexico Press.
All rights reserved.
First Edition.

Library of Congress
Cataloging-in-Publication Data

Racial and ethnic patterns of mortality in New
  Mexico/edited by Thomas M. Becker. . . .
  [et al.].
    p. cm.
  Includes bibliographical references and
index.
  ISBN 0–8263–1405–8
  1. Public health—New Mexico—
Statistics. 2. Indians of North America—
New Mexico—Health and hygiene.
3. Hispanic Americans—New Mexico—
Health and hygiene. I. Becker, Thomas M.
RA447.N7R3 1993
614.4′2789′089—dc20
                             92–29585
                                  CIP

Designed by Joanna V. Hill

Contents

List of Figures viii
List of Tables xii
Introduction xvii

1. **Methods** 1
   Death Certificate Data 1
   Ethnicity 1
   Population Estimates 2
   Age-Specific and Age-Adjusted Mortality Rates 8
   Age-Period-Cohort Graphs 8
   Coding Schemes of the International Classification of Diseases 9
   References 10

2. **All-Cause Mortality** 12
   Methodologic Considerations 12
   Results 12
   Discussion 14
   Summary 22
   References 22

3. **Cancer Mortality** 23
   Methodologic Considerations 24
   Results 24
   Discussion 38
   Summary 46
   References 47

4. **Diabetes Mortality** 50
   Methodologic Considerations 51
   Results 51
   Discussion 53
   Summary 61
   References 61

5. Infectious Diseases Mortality 65
Methodologic Considerations 65
Results 66
Discussion 66
Summary 78
Appendix 79
References 79

6. Ischemic Heart Disease Mortality 83
Methodologic Considerations 83
Results 84
Discussion 86
Summary 94
References 94

7. Respiratory Disease Mortality 98
Methodologic Considerations 99
Results 99
Discussion 100
Summary 104
References 105

8. Alcohol-Related Mortality 108
Methodologic Considerations 108
Results 109
Discussion 110
Summary 115
References 116

9. Injury Mortality 118
Methodologic Considerations 119
Results 119
Discussion 126
Summary 128
Appendix 129
References 129

10. Suicide and Homicide 132
Methodologic Considerations 132
Results 134

Discussion   136
Summary   141
References   141

11. Symptoms, Signs, and Ill-Defined Conditions: A Leading Cause of Death Among Minorities   145
Methodologic Considerations   146
Results   147
Discussion   150
Summary   158
References   158

12. Summary   160

Appendix: Average Annual Age-Adjusted Mortality Rates, New Mexico, 1958 through 1982   162

Index   227

Contributors   235

Figures

2.1 Mortality from all causes among non-Hispanic white males in New Mexico younger than 30 years, by 5-year birth cohort   15
2.2 Mortality from all causes among non-Hispanic white females in New Mexico younger than 30 years, by 5-year birth cohort   15
2.3 Mortality from all causes among Hispanic males in New Mexico younger than 30 years, by 5-year birth cohort   16
2.4 Mortality from all causes among Hispanic females in New Mexico younger than 30 years, by 5-year birth cohort   16
2.5 Mortality from all causes among American Indian males in New Mexico younger than 30 years, by 5-year birth cohort   17
2.6 Mortality from all causes among American Indian females in New Mexico younger than 30 years, by 5-year birth cohort   17
2.7 Mortality from all causes among non-Hispanic white males in New Mexico aged 30 years and older, by 5-year birth cohort   18
2.8 Mortality from all causes among non-Hispanic white females in New Mexico aged 30 years and older, by 5-year birth cohort   18
2.9 Mortality from all causes among Hispanic males in New Mexico aged 30 years and older, by 5-year birth cohort   19
2.10 Mortality from all causes among Hispanic females in New Mexico aged 30 years and older, by 5-year birth cohort   19
2.11 Mortality from all causes among American Indian males in New Mexico aged 30 years and older, by 5-year birth cohort   20
2.12 Mortality from all causes among American Indian females in New Mexico aged 30 years and older, by 5-year birth cohort   20

3.1 Stomach cancer mortality among non-Hispanic white males in New Mexico, by 5-year birth cohort   31
3.2 Stomach cancer mortality among non-Hispanic white females in New Mexico, by 5-year birth cohort   32
3.3 Stomach cancer mortality among Hispanic males in New Mexico, by 5-year birth cohort   33
3.4 Stomach cancer mortality among Hispanic females in New Mexico, by 5-year birth cohort   34
3.5 Colorectal cancer mortality among non-Hispanic white males in New Mexico, by 5-year birth cohort   35

FIGURES   ix

3.6   Colorectal cancer mortality among non-Hispanic white females in New Mexico, by 5-year birth cohort   36
3.7   Colorectal cancer mortality among Hispanic males in New Mexico, by 5-year birth cohort   37
3.8   Colorectal cancer mortality among Hispanic females in New Mexico, by 5-year birth cohort   38
3.9   Breast cancer mortality among non-Hispanic white females in New Mexico, by 5-year birth cohort   39
3.10   Breast cancer mortality among Hispanic females in New Mexico, by 5-year birth cohort   40

4.1   Diabetes mortality among non-Hispanic white males in New Mexico, by 5-year birth cohort   53
4.2   Diabetes mortality among non-Hispanic white females in New Mexico, by 5-year birth cohort   54
4.3   Diabetes mortality among Hispanic males in New Mexico, by 5-year birth cohort   55
4.4   Diabetes mortality among Hispanic females in New Mexico, by 5-year birth cohort   56
4.5   Multiple factors that affect the diabetes mortality rate   56

5.1   Pneumonia mortality among non-Hispanic white males in New Mexico, by 5-year birth cohort   69
5.2   Pneumonia mortality among non-Hispanic white females in New Mexico, by 5-year birth cohort   70
5.3   Pneumonia mortality among Hispanic males in New Mexico, by 5-year birth cohort   71
5.4   Pneumonia mortality among Hispanic females in New Mexico, by 5-year birth cohort   72
5.5   Pneumonia mortality among American Indian males in New Mexico, by 5-year birth cohort   73
5.6   Pneumonia mortality among American Indian females in New Mexico, by 5-year birth cohort   74
5.7   Tuberculosis mortality among American Indian males in New Mexico, by 5-year birth cohort   75
5.8   Tuberculosis mortality among American Indian females in New Mexico, by 5-year birth cohort   76

6.1   Ischemic heart disease mortality in non-Hispanic white males in New Mexico, by 5-year birth cohort   86
6.2   Ischemic heart disease mortality in non-Hispanic white females in New Mexico, by 5-year birth cohort   87

FIGURES

6.3 Ischemic heart disease mortality in Hispanic males in New Mexico, by 5-year birth cohort   88
6.4 Ischemic heart disease mortality in Hispanic females in New Mexico, by 5-year birth cohort   89
6.5 Ischemic heart disease mortality in American Indian males in New Mexico, by 5-year birth cohort   90
6.6 Ischemic heart disease mortality in American Indian females in New Mexico, by 5-year birth cohort   91

7.1 Lung cancer mortality in non-Hispanic white males in New Mexico, by 5-year birth cohort   101
7.2 Lung cancer mortality in non-Hispanic white females in New Mexico, by 5-year birth cohort   102
7.3 Lung cancer mortality in Hispanic males in New Mexico, by 5-year birth cohort   103
7.4 Lung cancer mortality in Hispanic females in New Mexico, by 5-year birth cohort   104

8.1 Alcohol-related mortality among non-Hispanic white males in New Mexico, by 5-year birth cohort   111
8.2 Alcohol-related mortality among non-Hispanic white females in New Mexico, by 5-year birth cohort   112
8.3 Alcohol-related mortality among Hispanic males in New Mexico, by 5-year birth cohort   113
8.4 Alcohol-related mortality among Hispanic females in New Mexico, by 5-year birth cohort   114
8.5 Alcohol-related mortality among American Indian males in New Mexico, by 5-year birth cohort   115
8.6 Alcohol-related mortality among American Indian females in New Mexico, by 5-year birth cohort   116

11.1 Mortality from symptoms, signs, and ill-defined conditions among non-Hispanic white males in New Mexico, by 5-year birth cohort   149
11.2 Mortality from symptoms, signs, and ill-defined conditions among non-Hispanic white females in New Mexico, by 5-year birth cohort   150
11.3 Mortality from symptoms, signs, and ill-defined conditions among Hispanic males in New Mexico, by 5-year birth cohort   151
11.4 Mortality from symptoms, signs, and ill-defined conditions among Hispanic females in New Mexico, by 5-year birth cohort   152
11.5 Mortality from symptoms, signs, and ill-defined conditions among

American Indian males in New Mexico, by 5-year birth cohort 153

11.6 Mortality from symptoms, signs, and ill-defined conditions among American Indian females in New Mexico, by 5-year birth cohort 154

Tables

1.1 Ethnic identifiers from the 1960, 1970, and 1980 U.S. censuses, and corresponding estimates of the Hispanic population   3
1.2 Age distribution of respondents by ethnicity and sex   5
1.3 Sensitivity and specificity of selected ethnic identifiers in comparison with the 1980 Spanish-origin question   5

2.1 Mortality rates in New Mexicans from all causes combined, by time period, age, and ethnicity, 1958 through 1982   13

3.1 Categories for selected malignant neoplasms, and corresponding codes in the seventh, eighth, and ninth revisions of the International Classification of Diseases   24
3.2 Cancer mortality rates in New Mexican males, U.S. white males, and U.S. black males by selected cancer primary sites, 1958 through 1982   25
3.3 Cancer mortality rates in New Mexican females, U.S. white females, and U.S. black females by selected cancer primary sites, 1958 through 1982   28

4.1 Diabetes mortality rates in New Mexican males and U.S. white males, 1958 through 1982   52
4.2 Diabetes mortality rates in New Mexican females and U.S. white females, 1958 through 1982   52

5.1 Infection-related mortality rates in New Mexican males by cause and ethnic group, 1958 through 1982   67
5.2 Infection-related mortality rates in New Mexican females by cause and ethnic group, 1958 through 1982   68
5.3 Infection-related mortality rates in New Mexican children aged 0 through 4 years by cause and ethnic group, 1958 through 1982   77

6.1 Mortality rates in New Mexicans from ischemic heart disease, 1958 through 1982   85

TABLES

7.1 Mortality rates in New Mexican males and U.S. white males from lung cancer and chronic obstructive pulmonary disease (COPD), 1958 through 1982   100

7.2 Mortality rates in New Mexican females and U.S. white females from lung cancer and chronic obstructive pulmonary disease (COPD), 1958 through 1982   105

8.1 Alcohol-related categories, and corresponding codes in the seventh, eighth, and ninth revisions of the International Classification of Diseases   109

8.2 Alcohol-related mortality rates in New Mexicans by ethnic group and sex, 1958 through 1982   110

9.1 Mortality rates in New Mexican males from total external causes, motor vehicle accidents, suicide, and homicide, as compared with selected U.S. rates, 1958 through 1982   120

9.2 Mortality rates in New Mexican females from total external causes, motor vehicle accidents, suicide, and homicide, as compared with selected U.S. rates, 1958 through 1982   121

9.3 Leading causes of injury mortality in American Indian, Hispanic, and non-Hispanic white males in New Mexico, 1958 through 1982   122

9.4 Leading causes of injury mortality in American Indian, Hispanic, and non-Hispanic white females in New Mexico, 1958 through 1982   123

10.1 Published suicide rates for American Indian tribes   133

10.2 Suicide rates in New Mexican Hispanics, American Indians, and non-Hispanic whites, 1958 through 1982   134

10.3 Age-specific suicide rates in New Mexican non-Hispanic white, Hispanic, and American Indian males, 1958 through 1982   135

10.4 Homicide rates in New Mexican Hispanics, American Indians, and non-Hispanic whites, 1958 through 1982   136

10.5 Age-specific homicide rates in New Mexican Hispanic, American Indian, and non-Hispanic white males, 1958 through 1982   137

11.1 Crude death rates from symptoms, signs, and ill-defined conditions for leading states, 1980   146

11.2 Mortality rates in New Mexicans from symptoms, signs, and ill-defined conditions, by ethnic group and sex, 1958 through 1982   148

11.3 Variation in ischemic heart disease mortality rates in New Mexicans, adjusted by the addition of mortality from symptoms, signs, and ill-defined conditions, 1978 through 1982   155

11.4 Variation in ischemic heart disease mortality rates in elderly New Mexicans, adjusted by the addition of mortality from symptoms, signs, and ill-defined conditions, 1978 through 1982   156

Acknowledgments

We thank Anthony Ortiz of the Bureau of Vital Statistics, Public Health Department, State of New Mexico, for data tapes used in these analyses. Without his consistent hard work and the assistance of his staff, this monograph would not have been possible. We also thank Dr. Cheryl Howard for her work in developing the ethnic-specific denominators for mortality rate calculations for this text, Mark Harty for preparing the graphics for publication, and Dorothy Fordyce for her patience and many hours of work transcribing the numerous revisions of the chapters.

Portions of this text originally appeared in earlier form in medical journals, and are reprinted here with permission. Portions of Chapter 5 appeared in the *American Journal of Public Health* 78 (1988) and 80 (1990), portions of Chapter 6 in *Circulation* 78 (1988), portions of Chapter 9 in the *Western Journal of Medicine* 150 (1989), portions of Chapter 10 in *Suicide and Life Threatening Behaviors* 20 (1990), and portions of Chapter 11 in the *American Journal of Epidemiology* 131 (1989).

This research was supported by the Flinn Foundation, Phoenix, Arizona, and by the National Cancer Institute through a contract with the Cancer Statistics Branch, which funds the New Mexico Tumor Registry. Initial development of the denominator estimates was supported by the U.S. Department of Energy, Office of Energy Research, under Grant No. DE-FG04-90ER60950.

Introduction

Thomas M. Becker
Rita S. Elliot

New Mexico is a state rich in the diversity of its colors, geography, architecture, and economy—and most outstanding of all—the diversity of its peoples and their cultures. New Mexico has a higher percentage of Hispanics and American Indians than any other state in the country. The Hispanic and American Indian peoples of New Mexico still hold to many cultural traditions that are apparent in their different lifestyles and everyday living and in their centuries-old festivals. According to the 1980 U.S. Census, 37% of the state's population are Hispanics and 8% are American Indians; of the remaining 55%, aproximately 2% are blacks or other minorities, and the rest are non-Hispanic whites. The U.S. Census of 1990 showed similar figures.

From a medical and epidemiologic point of view, the diversity of peoples and lifestyles in New Mexico presents a unique opportunity to study the ethnic distributions and risk factors for many diseases. Each of the predominant ethnic populations in the state has its own health and disease characteristics, which often differ substantially from the national norms for those characteristics. For various diseases, extreme differences are observed in rates of occurrence among the state's Hispanics, American Indians, and non-Hispanic whites. Differences in rates of morbidity and mortality among the state's ethnic groups may, in part, reflect genetic differences in host susceptibility. Rate differences for certain infections and chronic diseases may also reflect economic and cultural differences, such as differences in access to health care linked to economic status; the choice of health care other than that commonly provided by physicians and clinics, such as the services of medicine men, *curanderos* and *curanderas,* or herbalists; and different perceptions and understanding of the symptoms or signs of disease. The geography of New Mexico can also affect access to health care, and thus influence rates of morbidity and mortality for the many people in the state who live in remote areas where travel on unpaved roads is difficult or even impossible for part of the year.

With economic development and changes in health care resources and delivery, the health care problems of New Mexico have changed over the past quarter century. This monograph presents a summary of the changes in the health and disease profiles in New Mexico for the 25-year period 1958 through 1982 as observed through examination of statewide mortality data. The chapters summarize the time trends in mortality for major infectious and chronic diseases and injuries, with age, sex, and ethnic differences considered in the various analyses.

The information summarized in this text documents progress in providing health care to the people of New Mexico and suggests specific health-related problems that need to be addressed more aggressively. The book should prove useful to health care planners and to scholars interested in geographic medicine, epidemiology, or public health.

Readers who wish additional information on the histories of the diverse peoples of New Mexico are referred to the bibliography below for guidance. The text by J. L. Williams, *New Mexico in Maps*, is particularly useful for its insight into health-related problems in the state in addition to historical and demographic information about its peoples.

SELECTED BIBLIOGRAPHY

Dozier, E. P. *The Pueblo Indians of North America*. New York: Holt, Rinehart and Winston, Inc., 1970.

Ellis, R. N. *New Mexico Past and Present: A Historical Reader*. Albuquerque: University of New Mexico Press, 1971.

Fergusson, E. *New Mexico: A Pageant of Three Peoples*. Albuquerque: University of New Mexico Press, 1971.

Gonzalez, N. L. *The Spanish-Americans of New Mexico*. Albuquerque: University of New Mexico Press, 1971.

Kluckhohn, C., and D. Leighton. *The Navajo*. Garden City: Doubleday & Company, 1962.

Ortiz, A. *New Perspective on the Pueblos*. Albuquerque: University of New Mexico Press, 1972.

Ortiz, A., ed. *Handbook of North American Indians*. Vol. 9: *Southwest*. Washington, DC: Smithsonian Institution, 1979.

Roberts. S. A., and C. A. Roberts, *New Mexico*. Albuquerque: University of New Mexico Press, 1988.

Williams, J. L, ed. *New Mexico in Maps*. Albuquerque: University of New Mexico Press, 1986.

CHAPTER 1

Methods

Charles L. Wiggins
Jonathan M. Samet

This chapter presents the methods used in our research to (1) define the ethnic status of decedents, (2) determine ethnic group-specific denominators, (3) calculate death rates, and (4) identify specific causes of death by the categories used in the different volumes of the International Classification of Diseases (World Health Organization [WHO] 1957, 1967, 1977).

Death Certificate Data

We obtained coded death certificate data for New Mexico residents for the 25-year period 1958 through 1982 from the Vital Statistics Section of the New Mexico Health and Environment Department, Public Health Division. Cause of death was coded according to the seventh revision of the International Classification of Diseases (ICD) for 1958 through 1968 (WHO 1955), eighth ICD revision for 1969 through 1978 (WHO 1967), and the ninth ICD revision for 1979 through 1982 (WHO 1977).

Ethnicity

Ethnicity was assigned by the Bureau of Vital Statistics on the basis of information on individual death certificates. Hispanic ethnicity was determined on the basis of the decedents' surnames and the surnames of the decedents' parents, and from specific statements on the death certificate. American Indians were identified by death certificate designation. Non-Hispanic whites were individuals whose race was coded as white but who were not designated as Hispanic.

To validate this approach for designating ethnicity, we compared ethnicity as coded from the death certificate with that reported by subjects or next of kin for participants in a statewide case-control study conducted from 1980 through 1982 (Humble et al. 1985). Of the 222 cases and controls who identified themselves as Hispanic, 216 (97%) were classified as Hispanic by the Bureau of Vital Statistics. Of 291 non-Hispanic whites, only five (2%) were not similarly categorized by coding on the death certificate.

Population Estimates

Hispanics

The U.S. Census Bureau has attempted to enumerate the Hispanic population in each decennial census since 1930. The Bureau's methods of ethnic identification fall into two categories: objective and subjective. *Objective* ethnic identifiers rely on outward respondent characteristics, such as surname, language, birthplace, and parents' birthplace, that are linked with ethnic identity (Hernandez, Estrada, and Alvirez 1973). *Subjective* measures of ethnicity require the respondent to select or specify a meaningful group label that expresses his or her ethnic identity (Hernandez, Estrada, and Alvirez 1973). The Spanish-origin questions from the 1970 and 1980 censuses are examples of subjective Hispanic identifiers.

Changes with time in the outward characteristics of the Hispanic population may limit the accuracy of objective measures as ethnic identifiers. For example, birthplace is an unsatisfactory ethnic identifier for second- and third-generation Hispanics in the United States. Intermarriage with non-Hispanics reduces the validity of surname identifiers (Howard *et al.* 1983). Surname identifiers may also be affected by the current trend for married females to retain their maiden name rather than adopting their spouse's surname. In New Mexico and other southwestern states, American Indians with Spanish surnames could be classified as Hispanic if racial identifiers are not considered. Spanish-language use does not identify all Hispanics: 11.1 million people reported speaking Spanish at home in the 1980 Census, whereas the count for persons of Spanish origin was 14.6 million (David, Haub, and Willette 1983). Although subjective measures of ethnicity do not have the same limitations as objective identifiers, changes in concepts of ethnic identity and allegiance can vary both over time and among geographic areas (Siegel and Passel 1979).

We were confronted by potentially incomparable ethnic identifiers in calculating mortality rates for New Mexico Hispanics for the 25-year period 1958 through 1982 because the relevant censuses (1960, 1970, and 1980) offered Hispanic counts based on different techniques. In 1960, for example, ethnic identification based on surname relied on a list of Hispanic surnames that differed from the lists used in 1970 and 1980. Several different estimates of the state's Hispanic population were available from the 1970 Census (Table 1.1). In 1980, all households were

Table 1.1

Ethnic identifiers from the 1960, 1970, and 1980 U.S. censuses, and corresponding estimates of the Hispanic population

	United States	Five Southwestern States[a]	New Mexico
1960			
Spanish surname[b]	—	3,464,999	269,122
1970			
Spanish origin[c]	9,072,602	5,008,556	308,340
Spanish surname[d]			
(all races)	—	4,667,975	324,248
(white)	—	4,511,031	307,406
Spanish language[e]	9,589,216	5,662,700	379,723
Spanish heritage[f]	9,294,509	6,188,362	407,286
Birth and parentage[g]	5,241,892	2,321,642	40,173
1980			
Spanish origin[h]	14,608,673	8,787,795	477,222
Spanish surname[i]	—	7,746,347	432,850

[a] Arizona, California, Colorado, New Mexico, and Texas.

[b] White persons of Spanish surname according to the 1960 Census Bureau list, tabulated only for the five southwestern states.

[c] Self-identified Spanish origin, based on a 5% sample.

[d] Persons of Spanish surname according to the 1970 Census Bureau list, tabulated only for the five southwestern states.

[e] For the 1970 Census, all persons in a household where the head or wife reported "Spanish mother tongue" were included in the Spanish-language population.

[f] The Spanish-heritage population consists of persons of Spanish surname or language in the five southwestern states; persons of Puerto Rican birth or parentage in New York, New Jersey, and Pennsylvania; and persons of Spanish language in the remaining states and the District of Columbia.

[g] These data are based on the birthplace of the respondent and the birthplace(s) of his or her parents.

[h] Self-identified Spanish origin, based on a 100% sample.

[i] Persons of Spanish surname (all races) according to the 1980 Census Bureau list, tabulated only for the five southwestern states.

asked to supply information on Hispanic ethnicity, and an estimate of the Spanish-surnamed population was based on a sample of respondents. To understand better the comparability of the diverse identifiers used in the Censuses of 1960, 1970, and 1980, we conducted a survey of 1983 and 1984 to obtain information on the performance of these methods in a convenience sample of New Mexico Hispanics and non-Hispanics.

We assembled selected Census Bureau ethnic identifiers from the censuses of 1960, 1970, and 1980 into a single questionnaire. Questions concerning language, place of birth, Spanish origin, and race appeared on the questionnaire in the same language and format as on Census Bureau forms. Respondents were asked to record their own surname, their father's surname, their mother's maiden name, and the places of birth of both parents. To make completion of the questionnaire less monotonous and its intent less obvious, we interspersed the questions related to ethnicity among items unrelated to ethnicity. Respondents were also asked to list their sex, their year of birth, and the ZIP Code of their current place of residence.

To reach a large number of Hispanics at little cost, we distributed questionnaires to a convenience sample of adult New Mexico residents. Albuquerque respondents included University of New Mexico students and staff, senior citizens, and employees of Sandia National Laboratories. Questionnaires were also distributed among participants in the Albuquerque *Feria,* an annual celebration of Hispanic culture, and among recipients of services provided by the Home Education Livelihood Program. A group of respondents from Las Vegas, New Mexico, a largely Hispanic community located in the north-central portion of the state, was also included in the study. Because of the sampling methods, response rates were not calculated. For some analyses, respondents were classified as Hispanic or non-Hispanic based on their responses to the Spanish-origin question reproduced from the 1980 Census Bureau form. Ethnic classifications based on the remaining ethnic identifiers were then compared with responses to the 1980 Spanish-origin question. We assumed that a response to the 1980 Spanish-origin question represented the true ethnic identity, then for each of the remaining ethnic identifiers we calculated sensitivity, percentage of Hispanics correctly classified, and specificity, percentage of non-Hispanics correctly classified.

Respondent and parent surnames were classified as Hispanic or non-Hispanic based on the 1960, 1970, and 1980 Census Bureau lists of Spanish surnames. Surnames were classified in accordance with the rules and instructions that governed each list.

The survey included 6,643 subjects: 21% (n = 1,392) identified themselves as Hispanic on the 1980 Spanish-origin question, 73% (n = 4,848) identified themselves as non-Hispanic, and 6% (n = 403) did not respond to the question (Table 1.2).

With the 1980 Spanish-origin question as the standard for comparison, the 1970 Spanish-heritage and 1970 Spanish-origin identifiers had the highest sensitivity and specificity (Table 1.3). However, the similarly structured 1970 and 1980 Spanish-origin questions did not yield identi-

Table 1.2
Age distribution of respondents by ethnicity* and sex

	Hispanic		Non-Hispanic	
	Male (n = 617)	Female (n = 751)	Male (n = 2942)	Female (n = 1875)
Age Range (years)	*Percentage (%) of category*			
<20	6.3	3.7	0.2	0.4
20–29	19.1	25.7	10.2	15.9
30–39	25.0	25.4	22.0	26.8
40–49	17.7	13.8	27.3	18.9
50–59	14.4	11.3	24.4	15.2
60–69	9.9	10.7	12.3	13.1
70+	7.6	9.3	3.6	9.7

* Based on self-identified Spanish-origin question from the 1980 Census form. Total number of respondents: n = 6643. Table 1.2 is based on respondents who specified sex, birth year, and ethnicity.

Table 1.3
Sensitivity and specificity of selected ethnic identifiers in comparison with the 1980 Spanish-origin question

	Males		Females	
	Sensitivity	Specificity	Sensitivity	Specificity
	Percentage (%) of category			
1970 Spanish origin	93	100	91	99
1970 Spanish heritage	95	98	92	94
1970 Spanish language	91	98	86	96
1980 Census list of Spanish surnames	87	99	78	96
1970 Census list of Spanish surnames	84	99	74	96
1960 Census list of Spanish surnames	81	99	70	96

cal results. Lower sensitivity was observed for surname-based identifiers than for other methods, although the overall accuracy of the surname lists improved from 1960 through 1980. The sensitivity for each indicator was higher for males than for females and increased slightly with age of the respondent (age data not shown).

The results from our survey illustrate the extent of the differences among the various methods for classifying ethnicity. Discrepancies between a respondent's subjective ethnic identity and his or her objective outward characteristics account for many of these differences. In some instances, however, the same individual responded differently to similar subjective questions, as shown by respondents who called themselves "Hispanic" on the 1980 Spanish-origin question and "non-Hispanic" on the 1970 Spanish-origin question (Table 1.3). The Census Bureau has shown that relatively simple changes in wording or format can elicit different responses to similar questions (Fernandez and McKenney 1980).

We used the results of our survey to adjust estimates of New Mexico's Hispanic population as enumerated in the censuses of 1960 and 1970. The high concordance between responses to the 1980 Spanish-origin question and the 1970 Spanish-heritage identifier led us to choose the latter figures as the base estimates of the 1970 New Mexico Hispanic population; however, because the total Spanish-heritage population included people of all racial groups, we subtracted American Indians with Spanish surnames. Because we found low concordance between the 1960 Census Bureau list of Spanish surnames and the responses to the 1980 Spanish-origin identifier (Table 1.3), we upwardly adjusted estimates of New Mexico's Spanish-surnamed population from the 1960 census by dividing the number of Hispanic men and women by 0.81 and 0.70, respectively. These figures represent the sensitivity of the 1960 Spanish-surname list compared with self-reported responses to the 1980 Spanish-origin questions. Because the sensitivity did not vary by age, the adjustment factors were applied uniformly across all age strata.

In the 1980 U.S. Census, approximately 14% of New Mexico residents indicated that their race was "race not elsewhere classified" (not white, black, Indian, or Asian). On closer inspection, we found that 36% of those who identified themselves as Hispanic according to the 1980 Spanish-origin question also classified their race as "other" (not white, black, or Asian). The Census Bureau later determined that the majority of these individuals, by the Census Bureau definition, belonged in one of the traditional racial categories, and most were considered to be white. Because this misclassification (by census definition) occurred nationwide, corrections in the census data were needed for accurate calculation of vital statistics by ethnic group. The Census Bureau, under contract to the National Cancer Institute (NCI), arranged to correct systematically the errors in the population data for areas covered by the NCI's Surveillance, Epidemiology, and End Results (SEER) Program. The Hispanic population estimates for 1980 in New Mexico, one of 10 participants in the SEER Program, were corrected (Irwin 1983).

American Indians

The Census Bureau underestimated the size of the American Indian population in 1970 (Passel 1976). Although not documented, similar undercounts probably occurred in 1960 and in 1980. In lieu of more accurate data, and with the exception of specific adjustments outlined below, we have used census estimates of the American Indian population as published by the Census Bureau. Akers and Larmon (1967) reported that "smudges" on Census Bureau forms were read by optical scanning devices, thereby producing erroneous counts of American Indians in certain age groups in the 1960 census. Fortunately, Akers and Larmon also published correction factors for these errors, which we used to correct the Bureau's 1960 estimates of New Mexico's American Indian population.

Intercensal Estimates of New Mexico's Population

Annual estimates of New Mexico's total population are available for the years 1958 through 1959 (Bureau of Business and Economic Research 1984), 1961 through 1969 (Bureau of Business and Economic Research 1984), 1971 through 1979 (Irwin 1983), and 1981 through 1982 (U.S. Department of Commerce 1985). However, these intercensal estimates are for the population as a whole and are not distributed by age, gender, and racial and/or ethnic group. Because mortality rates vary by the latter three variables, it was necessary to estimate the detailed distribution of New Mexico's population to calculate accurate mortality rates.

We derived detailed estimates of New Mexico's population for years outside of the decennial censuses from proportional changes in the age, racial and/or ethnic, and gender distributions that occurred from one census to the next (using adjusted figures). Specifically, we calculated the proportion of the total New Mexico population in 1960, 1970, and 1980 that existed within each 5-year age group, gender, and racial and/or ethnic group. We applied the following linear model to annual midyear estimates of the total New Mexico population to estimate the age, gender, and racial and/or ethnic distribution for each intercensal year:

$$P_i = (B_{0,i} + [B_{1,i} I]) \, CT$$

where:

P_i = the race/ethnic-gender population in the ith age group at time x

$B_{0,i}$ = the proportion of the total New Mexico population in the ith age category in the index census

$B_{1,i}$ = the average annual rate of change in proportion to the population in the ith race/ethnic-gender group

I = the time interval (in years) from the index census to time x

CT = Census estimate of the total New Mexico population at time x

Estimates of New Mexico's total statewide population for 1958 and 1959 were distributed according to the same age, gender, and racial and/or ethnic distribution as our adjusted figures for 1960. Estimates of New Mexico's total statewide population for the years 1981 and 1982 were similarly distributed according to our adjusted population figures for 1980.

Age-Specific and Age-Adjusted Mortality Rates

We calculated age-specific and age-adjusted mortality rates for the 5-year periods 1958 through 1962, 1963 thorugh 1967, 1968 through 1972, 1973 through 1977, and 1978 through 1982. Age-adjusted mortality rates were calculated by the direct method (Rothman 1986) and were standardized to the distribution of the United States white population as enumerated in the 1970 U.S. Census (Cutler and Young 1975).

Throughout this monograph, we present age-specific and age-adjusted mortality rates among the state's three predominant ethnic groups. Age-specific mortality rates, usually presented by 5-year age groups, allow a valid comparison of mortality rates among the three major ethnic groups in the state. However, because the age structure of each of the state's major ethnic groups differs substantially, any comparison of crude mortality rates among New Mexico's ethnic populations would be misleading. For this reason, we have adjusted the cause-specific mortality rates for each ethnic group to a standard (or reference) population.

The calculation of an age-adjusted rate using the direct method (Rothman 1986) requires the age-specific rates in the population under study (American Indians, Hispanics, or non-Hispanic whites), and the population distribution of some standard population, such as the national standard population distribution during a specified year. For our age-adjusted rate calculations, we used the distribution of the U.S. white population as enumerated in the 1970 U.S. Census (Cutler and Young 1975). Calculation of an age-adjusted rate removes the effect of age differential, and so allows a meaningful comparison of cause-specific mortality. This technique is a standard practice worldwide among epidemiologists, demographers, and other social scientists.

Age-Period-Cohort Graphs

In several of the chapters in this monograph, we present mortality trend data in the form of age-period-cohort graphs. Such graphical presentations reflect changes in cause-specific mortality rates by age group and birth cohort. Period effects, which can reflect technological changes in disease diagnosis or treatment, can also be determined from these graphs.

Although such graphs are useful to present changes in mortality by age, by birth cohort, or by period, the confounding of these effects limits one's ability to identify which factor or factors exert the strongest influence in changing mortality rates (Glenn 1977). We have included such graphs only when trends in cause-specific mortality were of sufficient magnitude to warrant graphical display.

Coding Schemes of the International Classification of Diseases

The International Classification of Diseases (ICD) codes for specific causes of death have changed over the 25-year period of our study, 1958 through 1982. For example, for ischemic heart disease, the codes changed substantially from the seventh revision of the ICD (1958 through 1968) to the eighth revision (1969 through 1978), and changed again in the ninth revision. Because of the changes in coding schemes among the various ICD revisions, we adjusted the numerators for cause-specific mortality for specific causes of death employing ICD comparability ratios (U.S. Department of Health, Education, and Welfare 1968, 1980). For example, for ischemic heart disease, we adjusted all deaths recorded over the 25-year period to the coding scheme of the eighth ICD revision. Changes in coding procedures for ischemic heart disease in 1969 resulted in the assignment of more deaths to this category than had been assigned to the most nearly comparable category ("arteriosclerotic heart disease, including coronary artery disease") in the seventh revision (U.S. Department of Health, Education, and Welfare 1979). The resulting comparability ratio of 1.146 expresses the differences in coding changes between the seventh and eighth ICD revisions. A comparability ratio of 0.998 results if ischemic heart disease (ICD 410-413, eighth revision) is compared with the following combined categories in the ICD seventh revision: "arteriosclerotic heart disease, including coronary disease" (ICD 420), and "other hypertensive heart disease" (ICD 440, 441, and 443) (U.S. Department of Health, Education, and Welfare 1979). We also adjusted the mortality figures for 1979 through 1982, coded under the ninth ICD revision, to make them more comparable with data coded under the eighth ICD revision for ischemic heart disease.

In this monograph, we indicate coding changes and data that have been adjusted by employing comparability ratios. When not otherwise indicated, the data are presented unadjusted for changes in the ICD coding schemes. For further discussion of comparability ratios, readers may consult the monthly Vital Statistics Reports from the National Center for Health Statistics (U.S. Department of Health, Education, and Welfare 1968, 1980).

REFERENCES

Akers, D. S., and E. A. Larmon. 1967. Indians and smudges on the census schedule. In *Proc.Soc.Stat.Sect.; Am.Stat.Assoc.1967*: 369–73. Washington, DC: The American Statistical Association.
Bureau of Business and Economic Research, Institute for Applied Research Services. New Mexico Statistical Services. 1984. *New Mexico Statistical Abstract, 1984*. Albuquerque, NM: University of New Mexico Press.
Cutler, S. J., and J. L. Young, Jr., eds. 1975. *Third national cancer survey: incidence data* (p. 449). National Cancer Institute Monograph 41. DHEW Publication No. (NIH) 75–787. Washington, DC: U.S. Government Printing Office.
David, C., C. Haub, and J. Willette. 1983. U.S. Hispanics: changing the face of America. *Population Bulletin* 38:1–44.
Fernandez, E. W., and N. R. McKenney, 1980. *Identification of the Hispanic population: a review of Census Bureau experiences*. Washington, DC: U.S. Bureau of the Census, Population Division.
Glenn, N. D. 1977. Cohort analysis. In G. Iversen and H. Norpoln. *Analysis of variance*. Beverly Hills: Sage Publications.
Hernandez, J., L. Estrada, and D. Alvirez. 1973. Census data and the problem of conceptually defining the Mexican American population. *Soc. Sci. Q.* 53: 671–87.
Howard, C. A., J. M. Samet, R. W. Buechley, S. D. Schrag, and C. R. Key. 1983. Survey research in New Mexico Hispanics: some methodological issues. *Am.J. Epidemiol.* 117:27–34.
Humble, C. G., J. M. Samet, D. R. Pathak, and B. J. Skipper. 1985. Cigarette smoking in "Hispanic" whites and other whites in New Mexico. *Am.J.Public Health* 75:145–8.
Irwin, D. 1983. Bureau of the Census contract work for the National Cancer Institute's Surveillance, Epidemiology, and End Results Program.
Passel, J. S. 1976. Provisional evaluation of the 1970 census count of American Indians. *Demography* 13:397–409.
Rothman, K. J. 1986. *Modern epidemiology*. Boston/Toronto: Little, Brown, and Company.
Siegel, J. S., and J. S. Passel. 1979. *Coverage of the Hispanic population of the United States in the 1970 Census: a methodological analysis*. Current population reports, special studies P-23, No. 82. Washington, DC: U.S. Government Printing Office.
U.S. Department of Commerce, Bureau of the Census. 1985. *Estimates of the population of New Mexico counties and metropolitan areas: July 1, 1981, 1982, and 1983*. Series P-26, No. 83-31-C. Washington, DC: U.S. Government Printing Office.
U.S. Department of Health, Education, and Welfare. 1968. *Provisional estimates of selected comparability ratios*. Washington, DC: U.S. Government Printing Office.

———. 1979. *Proceedings of the Conference on the Decline in Coronary Heart Mortality.* Washington, DC: U.S. Government Printing Office.

———. 1980. *Estimates of selected comparability ratios.* Washington, DC: U.S. Government Printing Office.

World Health Organization. 1957. *Manual of the International Statistical Classification of Diseases, Injuries, and Causes of Death.* Based on the recommendations of the Seventh Revision Conference, 1955. Geneva, Switzerland: WHO.

———. 1967. *Manual of the International Statistical Classification of Diseases, Injuries, and Causes of Death.* Based on the recommendations of the Eighth Revision Conference. Geneva, Switzerland: WHO.

———. 1977. *Manual of the International Statistical Classification of Diseases, Injuries, and Causes of Death.* Based on the recommendations of the Ninth Revision Conference. Geneva, Switzerland: WHO.

CHAPTER 2

All-Cause Mortality

David K. Espey
Jonathan M. Samet
Charles L. Wiggins
Thomas M. Becker

Consideration of mortality from all causes of death combined provides a broad and essential perspective on the health of a population. If we assume complete death registration, all-cause mortality is not influenced by the factors that can affect cause-specific mortality. Thus, examination of all-cause mortality rates among New Mexico's racial and ethnic groups provides a comparison of health status that may be unbiased by differences among the populations in health care utilization, residence location, and other factors. To examine trends in all-cause mortality in New Mexico for the years 1958 through 1982, we compared age-specific mortality rates among the state's three main ethnic groups. We found distinct ethnic-specific, age-specific, and sex-specific trends in all-cause mortality among the state's American Indians, Hispanics, and non-Hispanic whites. The disparities among ethnic groups for ages younger than 45 years were particularly striking. In this age group, American Indian mortality rates among males were consistently 1.5 to 3 times that of non-Hispanic white males. In older age groups (65 years and greater), mortality rates were generally higher for non-Hispanic whites.

Methodologic Considerations

We combined all causes of death from the New Mexico Bureau of Vital Statistics tapes over the 25-year period 1958 through 1982.

Results

All-cause mortality rates in New Mexico from 1958 through 1982 revealed distinct patterns by ethnicity and sex (Table 2.1). Male mortality

Table 2.1

Mortality rates* in New Mexicans from all causes combined, by time period, age, and ethnicity, 1958 through 1982

	Time period (inclusive years)				
	1958–62	1963–67	1968–72	1973–77	1978–82
Males					
Non-Hispanic white	1,086.8	1,054.4	1,097.2	1,066.0	964.1
	(11,162)[a]	(12,426)	(12,995)	(14,475)	(15,755)
Hispanic	953.4	968.8	1,036.5	951.3	922.2
	(6,082)	(6,384)	(6,975)	(7,138)	(7,627)
American Indian	1,098.9	1,111.9	1,332.9	1,494.5	1,153.2
	(1,338)	(1,526)	(1,797)	(2,247)	(2,006)
U.S. white	1,207.0	1,188.2	1,176.0	1,084.1	1,004.7
U.S. black	1,508.2	1,530.7	1,571.6	1,424.8	1,374.0
Females					
Non-Hispanic white	607.7	542.5	609.5	604.1	561.8
	(7,101)	(7,855)	(9,045)	(10,387)	(11,984)
Hispanic	698.9	648.8	676.5	596.2	531.6
	(4,367)	(4,403)	(4,511)	(4,448)	(4,650)
American Indian	671.4	759.8	798.1	742.3	622.6
	(857)	(1,062)	(1,086)	(1,116)	(1,062)
U.S. white	777.4	737.0	700.1	632.5	597.3
U.S. black	1,119.8	1,060.8	1,011.6	881.2	823.2

* Age-adjusted rates per 100,000.
[a] Numbers of deaths are given in parentheses.

was consistently higher in all age groups regardless of ethnicity. For both sexes, all-cause mortality was highest in American Indians.

Age-period-cohort graphs (Figures 2.1 through 2.12) display mortality over time by age, sex, and ethnic group. In the youngest age group, 0 through 4 years, all-cause mortality reflects primarily infant mortality. The mortality rates decreased for all ethnic groups from 1958 through 1982, but most dramatically for American Indians. At the beginning of the study period, American Indian mortality for this 0-through-4 age group was twice that of non-Hispanic whites. Over the study period, the rates for American Indians were more than halved, but remained substantially greater than for non-Hispanic whites. Mortality for Hispanics was intermediate, although closer to that of non-Hispanic whites by the end of the study period.

For the age groups 5 through 14 years, mortality was lowest and generally showed a decline over the course of study for all groups except American Indian males, who initially showed a marked relative rise. For age groups 15 through 24 years, 25 through 34 years, and 35 through 44 years, American Indian males had the highest rates and the greatest increase over the study period. Non-Hispanic and Hispanic females, with comparable rates, had the lowest. Hispanic males also had very high rates, with a notable rise during the study period.

For age groups 45 through 64 years, mortality rates in males were highest for American Indians, roughly 150% to 200% of those of non-Hispanic and Hispanic white males. This pattern was similar for females in this age group, with relative mortality rates roughly half those of males. By sex, rates for age groups 55 through 64 years tended to be comparable among ethnic groups.

For age groups 65 through 74 years and 75 years and older, mortality for males was greatest for non-Hispanic whites, intermediate for Hispanic whites, and lowest for American Indians. For females in the older age groups, Hispanics had higher mortality rates, followed by non-Hispanic whites and American Indians, though the pattern was less consistent than for males.

Discussion

All-cause mortality rates of a population integrate the factors contributing to death in the population. By examining and comparing all-cause mortality rates among populations, we can describe general trends of health status and life expectancy. Improvements have been achieved in the study of mortality from specific causes by applying the International Classification of Diseases scheme, which is used to assign cause of death to each death certificate in the U.S. Use of this coding scheme has limitations, however. When cause of death is uncertain, general categories such as "symptoms, signs, and ill-defined conditions" are often used. Since uncertainty is more likely to exist in the absence of recent health care, it has been suggested that the use of this category may be an indicator of access to health care, and can introduce substantial bias into mortality rates for specific causes (Becker *et al.* 1990).

All-cause mortality is not subject to the vagaries of cause-of-death coding and therefore is a less biased, albeit more general, indicator of the health status of a population. By calculating and comparing mortality rates by age group, sex, and ethnic group, we can make correlations with known ethnic and age-specific morbidity and mortality.

The declining rates for all three ethnic groups in the age group 0

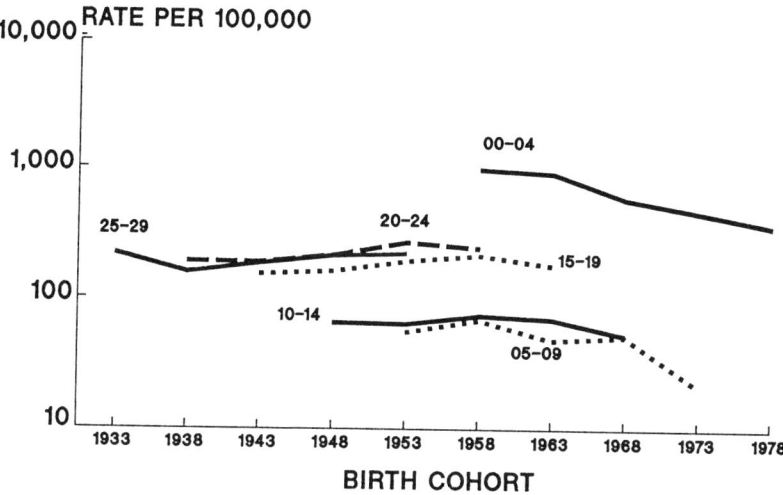

Figure 2.1. Mortality from all causes among non-Hispanic white males in New Mexico younger than 30 years, by 5-year birth cohort.

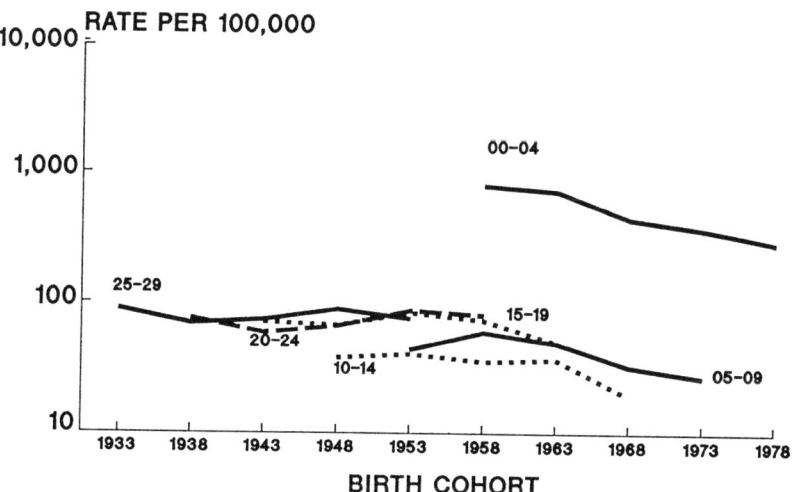

Figure 2.2. Mortality from all causes among non-Hispanic white females in New Mexico younger than 30 years, by 5-year birth cohort.

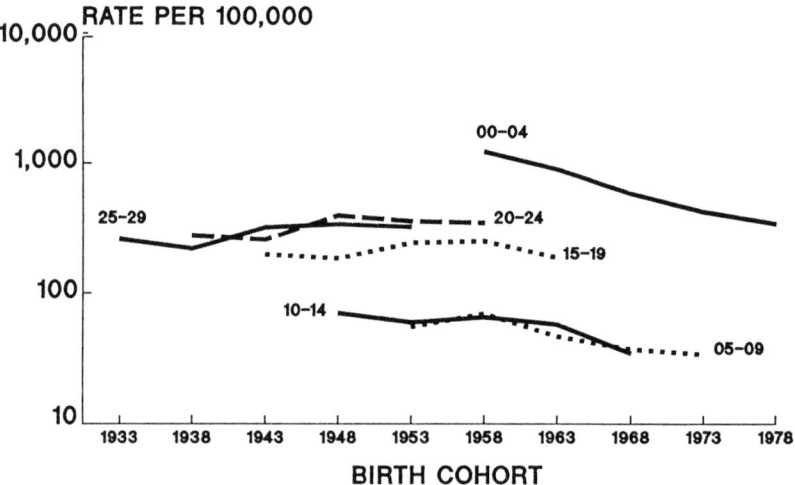

Figure 2.3. Mortality from all causes among Hispanic males in New Mexico younger than 30 years, by 5-year birth cohort.

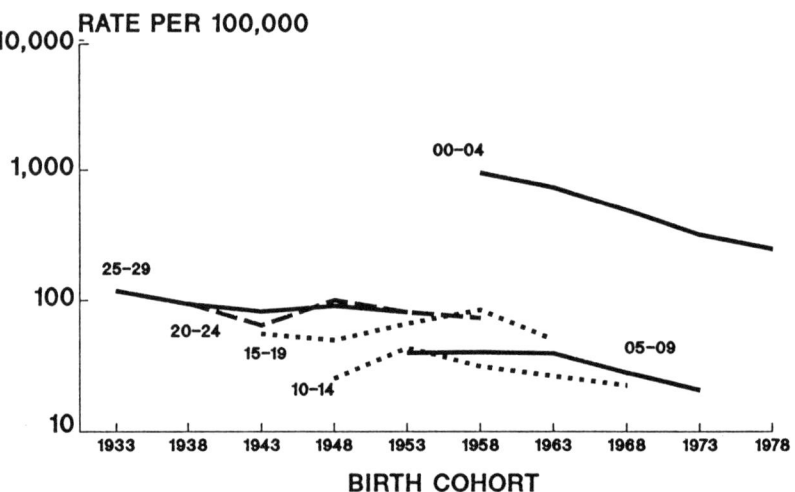

Figure 2.4. Mortality from all causes among Hispanic females in New Mexico younger than 30 years, by 5-year birth cohort.

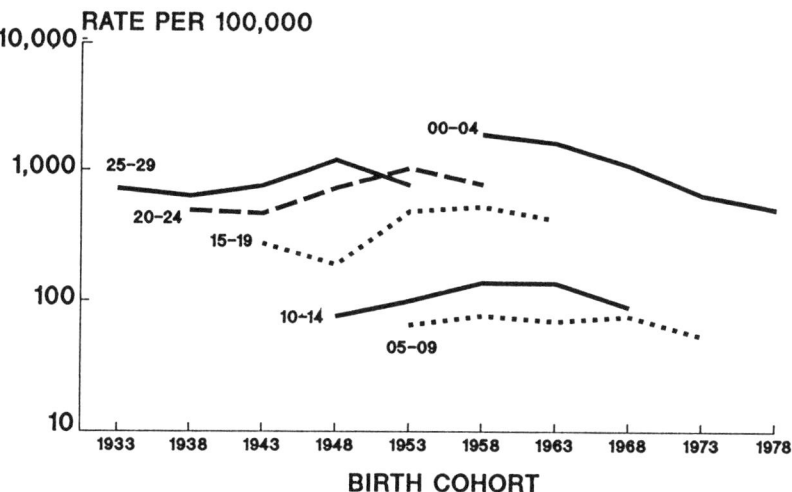

Figure 2.5. Mortality from all causes among American Indian males in New Mexico younger than 30 years, by 5-year birth cohort.

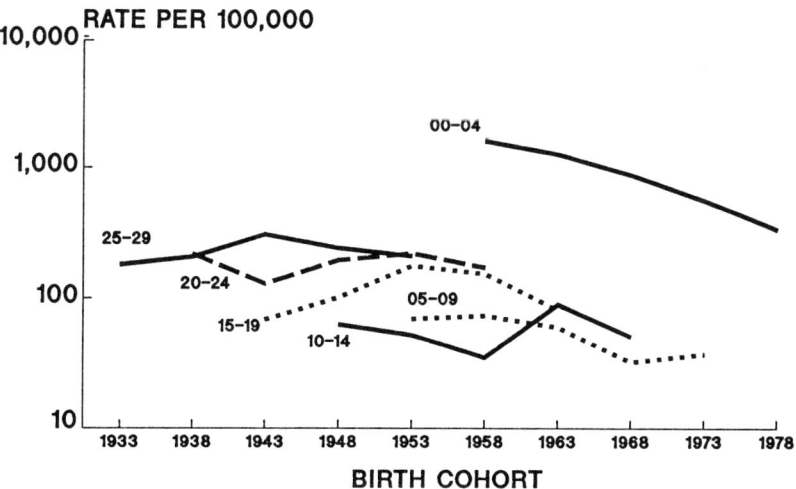

Figure 2.6. Mortality from all causes among American Indian females in New Mexico younger than 30 years, by 5-year birth cohort.

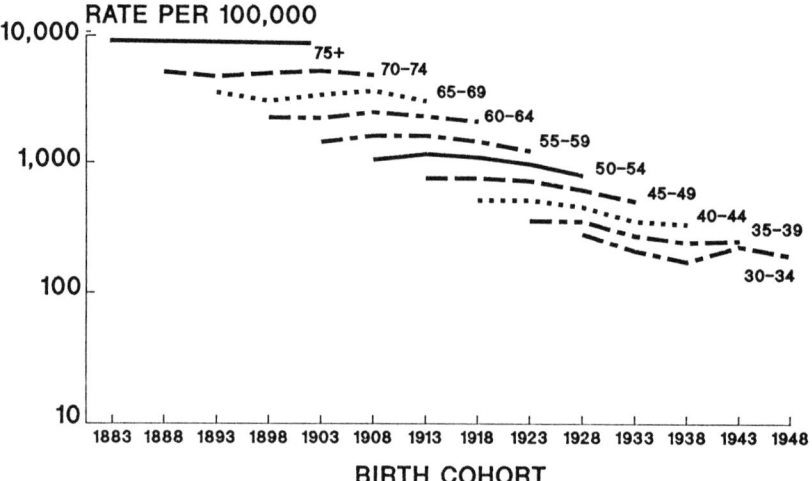

Figure 2.7. Mortality from all causes among non-Hispanic white males in New Mexico aged 30 years and older, by 5-year birth cohort.

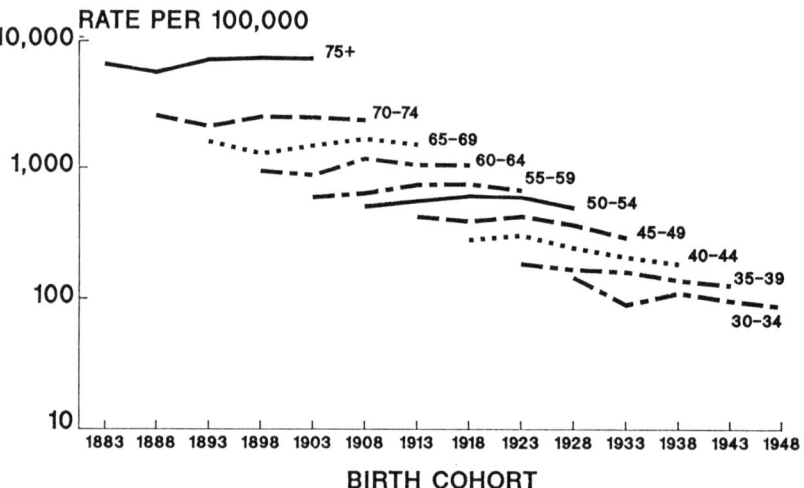

Figure 2.8. Mortality from all causes among non-Hispanic white females in New Mexico aged 30 years and older, by 5-year birth cohort.

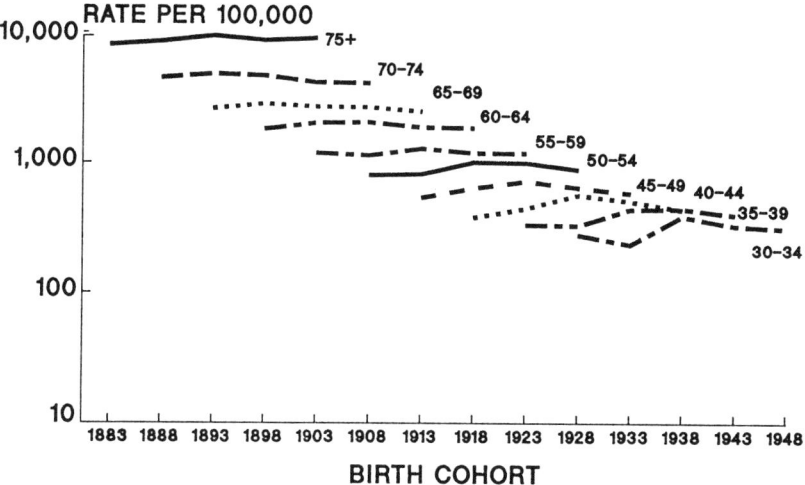

Figure 2.9. Mortality from all causes among Hispanic males in New Mexico aged 30 years and older, by 5-year birth cohort.

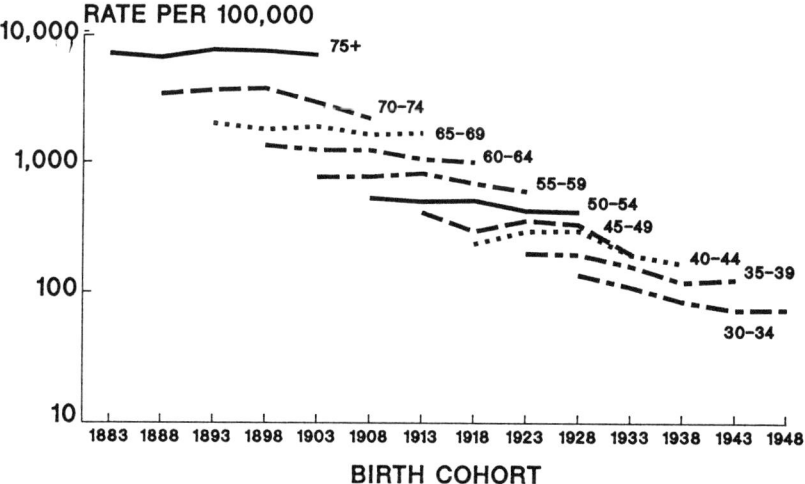

Figure 2.10. Mortality from all causes among Hispanic females in New Mexico aged 30 years and older, by 5-year birth cohort.

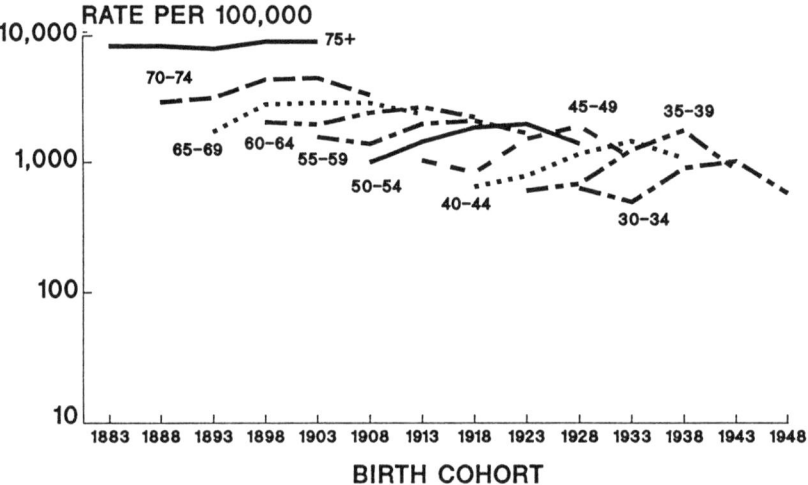

Figure 2.11. Mortality from all causes among American Indian males in New Mexico aged 30 years and older, by 5-year birth cohort.

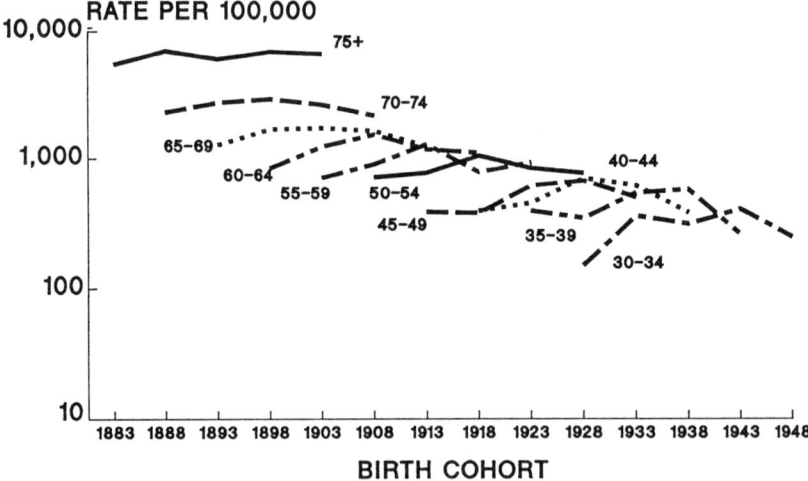

Figure 2.12. Mortality from all causes among American Indian females in New Mexico aged 30 years and older, by 5-year birth cohort.

through 4 years reflect the national downward trend of infant mortality during the study period. However, although the American Indian rate in New Mexico showed the greatest decline in the three ethnic groups, it remained substantially higher than the rates for Hispanic and non-Hispanic white children. The quality and availability of health care for American Indians improved dramatically with the establishment of the Indian Health Service, and the important decrease in infant mortality among American Indian babies must at least partially reflect improving prenatal care, immunizations, and treatment of infectious diseases. Nonetheless, a relatively high infant mortality rate persists among American Indian babies. This high infant mortality rate may be due to the large number of American Indians in the state who live below the poverty level and in remote isolated areas, two conditions that can seriously restrict access to clinical care (Rhoades, D'Angelo, and Ward 1987).

In the three age groups 15 through 24, 25 through 34, and 35 through 44, many deaths, especially among males, are the result of injuries of various types, and many are preventable (Sewell *et al.* 1989). The important differences in mortality between ethnic groups of young people in these age ranges have significant public and preventive health implications. Alcohol is a catalyst for injury and as such is a major source of mortality; however, the problem of alcohol is preventable, and so are most of the injuries (May 1986). Mortality and years of potential life lost could be reduced by orienting preventive and rehabilitative efforts towards the groups most affected by alcohol and other injury-related mortality. In New Mexico, the mortality data indicate the need to target Hispanic males and American Indian males and females.

In the age groups 45 through 54, and 55 through 64 years, injury plays a lesser role in mortality rates, while the major chronic diseases, particularly heart disease, assume increasing importance. In these age groups, the dramatic differences in mortality between the ethnic groups are less apparent.

The overall pattern in New Mexico of higher mortality rates in American Indians and Hispanics in the younger age groups and of lower mortality rates in the older age groups relative to non-Hispanic whites, can be related to known ethnic trends of disease and distribution of risk factors. Several chronic diseases that contribute greatly to overall mortality rates show distinct ethnic differences. For example, lung cancer and chronic obstructive pulmonary disease are common causes of death in non-Hispanic whites, are less common in Hispanics, and are infrequent in American Indians (Humble *et al.* 1985; Samet *et al.* 1988). These differences reflect differences in the level of consumption of cigarettes by the three ethnic groups in New Mexico. Because American Indians tend to smoke very little, these diseases are not important contributors to mortality in American Indians in New Mexico (Samet *et al.* 1988). Ischemic heart disease is also a leading cause of death for older individuals in all three ethnic groups. This disease also is most common among non-Hispanic whites, less common among Hispanic whites, and least common among American Indians.

Summary

All-cause mortality rates are a useful and readily available indicator of population health. All-cause mortality is not influenced by inconsistencies in coding schemes or access to health care, and it allows comparisons among populations to determine general levels of health status. In New Mexico for the years 1958 through 1982, general trends of higher mortality rates for Indian and Hispanic males in the younger age groups contrasted with lower rates in the older age groups, compared with the rates for non-Hispanic whites. We conclude that all-cause mortality rates are generally useful, and provide insights into culturally heterogeneous populations when examined by race, and by ethnicity, sex, and age.

REFERENCES

Becker, T. M., C. L. Wiggins, C. R. Key, and J. M. Samet. 1990. Symptoms, signs and ill-defined conditions: a leading cause of death among minorities. *Am.J. Epidemiol.* 131:664–8.

Humble, C. G., J. M. Samet, D. R. Pathak, and B. J. Skipper. 1985. Cigarette smoking and lung cancer in Hispanic whites and other whites in New Mexico. *Am.J.Public Health* 75:145–148.

May, P. 1986. Alcohol and drug misuse prevention programs for American Indians: needs and opportunities. *J.Stud.Alcohol* 47:187–195.

Rhoades, E. R., A. J. D'Angelo, and W. B. Ward. 1987. The Indian Health Service record of achievement. *Public Health Reports, July-August 1987.* 102(4):356.

Samet, J. M., C. L. Wiggins, C. R. Key, and T. M. Becker. 1988. Mortality from lung cancer and chronic obstructive pulmonary disease in New Mexico 1958–1982. *Am.J.Public Health* 78:1182–1186.

Sewell, C. M., T. M. Becker, C. L. Wiggins, C. R. Key, H. R. Hull, and J. M. Samet. 1989. Injury mortality in New Mexico's American Indians, Hispanics and non-Hispanic whites, 1958 to 1982. *West.J.Med.* 150:708–713.

CHAPTER 3

Cancer Mortality

Charles L. Wiggins
Thomas M. Becker
Charles R. Key
Jonathan M. Samet

Cancer mortality rates reflect both the underlying incidence rates of disease and the case-fatality rates. For cancers with high case-fatality rates, such as lung cancer, mortality and incidence rates are similar; as the case-fatality rate drops, the difference between incidence and mortality rates increases. For potentially curable cancers—for example, cervical cancer—mortality rates may be extremely low. Percy, Stanek, and Gloeckler (1981) have advised caution in interpreting cancer mortality rates. Determinants of the case-fatality rate are diverse and include medical factors such as the efficacy of treatment; and nonmedical factors such as access to treatment and delay in seeking treatment. Thus, differing mortality rates for cancer may be the result of differing incidence rates, of differing case-fatality rates, or of differences in both.

Racial and ethnic differences in cancer incidence and mortality rates in the United States are well documented (Horm et al. 1984). In the United States, cancer incidence is higher in blacks than whites, and is generally less common among persons of Hispanic, American Indian, and Asian ancestry. Cancer also occurs at different rates among the largest ethnic groups in New Mexico (Horm et al. 1984). With few exceptions, New Mexico's non-Hispanic whites exhibit cancer patterns similar to those of U.S. whites. In contrast, Hispanics are at approximately two-thirds the overall risk of developing cancer as are non-Hispanic whites, and American Indians are at approximately half the overall risk. However, on a site-by-site basis there are striking differences in the incidence of cancer among the three groups. The mortality rates described in this chapter supplement the incidence data routinely reported by the New Mexico Tumor Registry, and allow us to assess temporal changes in the occurrence of cancer in New Mexico during the 25-year period 1958 through 1982.

Table 3.1
Categories for selected malignant neoplasms, and corresponding codes in the seventh, eighth, and ninth revisions of the International Classification of Diseases

Cancer primary site	Codes		
	ICD7	ICD8	ICD9
Stomach	151	151	151
Colon and rectum	153–154	153–154	153–154
Pancreas	157	157	157
Trachea, bronchus, lung	162–163	162	162
Female breast	170	174	174
Cervix uteri	171	180	180
Corpus and other uterus	172–174	181–182	179, 181–182
Ovary, Fallopian tube, broad ligament	175	183	183
Prostate	177	185	185
Bladder	181	188	188
Brain and nervous system	193	191–192	191–192
Hodgkin's lymphoma	201	201	201
Leukemia	204	204–207	204–208

Methodologic Considerations

During the period of this study, deaths from malignant neoplasms were coded according to three revisions of the International Classification of Disease (ICD) (Table 3.1). The categories of malignant neoplasms were chosen, in part, to minimize bias caused by changes in disease classification. Because the term "cancer" represents a group of diseases rather than a single disease, and because the overall scope of malignant neoplasms changed somewhat between ICD revisions, we chose not to report rates for all sites combined. Rather, we selected for detailed discussion cancer sites that have a number of cases adequate to calculate stable rates for the ethnic groups within specific time intervals.

Results

Average annual age-adjusted cancer mortality rates for New Mexico males and females are shown in Tables 3.2 and 3.3. In the following paragraphs we discuss mortality patterns of selected cancers in the three

Table 3.2

Cancer mortality rates* in New Mexican males, U.S. white males, and U.S. black males by selected cancer primary sites, 1958 through 1982

Cancer primary site and ethnic group	Time period (inclusive years)				
	1958–62	1963–67	1968–72	1973–77	1978–82
Stomach					
NM non-Hispanic white	13.6	7.8	6.0	5.9	6.2
	(126)[a]	(91)	(69)	(80)	(103)
NM Hispanic	32.6	21.4	23.6	15.3	16.1
	(165)	(119)	(136)	(98)	(116)
NM American Indian	12.8	13.9	16.0	17.5	16.1
	(10)	(13)	(15)	(19)	(20)
U.S. white	16.2	12.5	10.4	8.8	7.6
U.S. black	26.0	22.6	20.0	17.4	14.6
Colon and rectum					
NM non-Hispanic white	15.4	14.4	20.0	20.4	22.8
	(152)	(168)	(232)	(279)	(368)
NM Hispanic	9.1	8.4	10.1	13.8	15.1
	(47)	(46)	(58)	(90)	(108)
NM American Indian	2.6	3.2	4.2	6.7	6.1
	(2)	(3)	(5)	(7)	(8)
U.S. white	25.5	25.7	25.6	25.8	25.3
U.S. black	18.8	20.4	22.5	24.2	26.4
Pancreas					
NM non-Hispanic white	7.1	10.1	9.9	9.0	10.5
	(70)	(120)	(121)	(127)	(178)
NM Hispanic	6.4	9.2	9.7	12.5	12.0
	(33)	(52)	(57)	(79)	(86)
NM American Indian	2.7	5.6	3.1	2.9	4.8
	(2)	(5)	(3)	(3)	(6)
U.S. white	10.1	10.8	11.2	11.0	10.3
U.S. black	10.7	13.3	12.8	14.0	13.8
Trachea, bronchus, lung					
NM non-Hispanic white	30.1	34.6	48.3	56.6	62.9
	(313)	(431)	(609)	(800)	(1073)
NM Hispanic	10.1	14.5	18.2	20.1	28.8
	(51)	(80)	(104)	(131)	(205)
NM American Indian	5.3	4.7	9.0	7.7	10.8
	(4)	(5)	(9)	(9)	(14)
U.S. white	38.5	47.5	57.8	64.8	70.4
U.S. black	38.0	48.0	66.1	80.4	93.4

Table 3.2 (*continued*)

Cancer primary site and ethnic group	1958–62	1963–67	1968–72	1973–77	1978–82
Prostate					
NM non-Hispanic white	18.6	15.9	18.4	19.8	25.4
	(157)	(170)	(199)	(250)	(388)
NM Hispanic	11.4	14.1	17.3	14.3	19.8
	(54)	(75)	(96)	(88)	(136)
NM American Indian	12.3	7.6	11.0	17.4	15.2
	(9)	(7)	(10)	(18)	(19)
U.S. white	19.2	19.2	19.3	20.2	21.1
U.S. black	31.8	33.2	37.3	41.2	44.3
Bladder					
NM non-Hispanic white	4.5	5.0	5.8	6.0	6.9
	(39)	(57)	(68)	(78)	(108)
NM Hispanic	2.1	1.2	2.3	3.0	3.7
	(10)	(6)	(13)	(19)	(26)
NM American Indian	1.2	0.0	1.1	0.9	0.0
	(1)	(0)	(1)	(1)	(0)
U.S. white	7.4	7.0	7.4	7.5	6.8
U.S. black	5.5	5.6	6.0	5.5	4.8
Brain					
NM non-Hispanic white	3.2	4.5	3.8	6.0	5.6
	(40)	(60)	(50)	(91)	(96)
NM Hispanic	1.6	2.7	1.8	3.4	4.2
	(12)	(20)	(12)	(27)	(36)
NM American Indian	1.7	0.4	3.2	1.7	1.5
	(2)	(1)	(3)	(3)	(2)
U.S. white	4.4	4.7	5.0	5.0	5.2
U.S. black	2.3	2.6	2.8	3.2	2.8
Hodgkin's lymphoma					
NM non-Hispanic white	1.5	2.9	2.1	1.5	0.8
	(18)	(39)	(29)	(23)	(15)
NM Hispanic	1.1	1.2	1.9	1.4	1.3
	(9)	(10)	(13)	(12)	(13)
NM American Indian	0.0	0.0	0.0	0.9	0.0
	(0)	(0)	(0)	(1)	(0)
U.S. white	2.3	2.4	2.2	1.5	1.1
U.S. black	1.6	1.7	1.9	1.3	1.0

Table 3.2 (*continued*)

Cancer primary site and ethnic group	Time period (inclusive years)				
	1958–62	1963–67	1968–72	1973–77	1978–82
Leukemia					
NM non-Hispanic white	7.8	9.4	7.8	8.5	8.9
	(83)	(111)	(93)	(116)	(152)
NM Hispanic	4.0	6.9	3.9	4.9	5.9
	(28)	(51)	(32)	(45)	(51)
NM American Indian	3.4	5.2	2.5	3.9	2.6
	(5)	(9)	(3)	(8)	(5)
U.S. white[b]	9.4	9.3	9.2	9.1	9.1
U.S. black[b]	5.4	6.6	7.4	7.2	7.4

*Age-adjusted rates per 100,000.
[a]Numbers of deaths are given in parentheses.
[b]Rates for U.S. whites and blacks are calculated for the midpoints of each 5-year interval (1960, 1965, 1970, 1975, 1980).

major ethnic groups in New Mexico for the years 1958 through 1982. Cancer of the lung is considered in a separate chapter.

Stomach

Age-standardized stomach cancer mortality rates for Hispanic and non-Hispanic whites declined from 1958 through 1982 (Tables 3.2 and 3.3), with a 50% reduction for Hispanics of both sexes and for non-Hispanic white males, and a 28% reduction for non-Hispanic white females. In contrast, rates were relatively stable for American Indians throughout the same period. Non-Hispanic whites were at a slightly lower risk of death from stomach cancer than were U.S. whites. Rates for New Mexico Hispanics were similar to those for U.S. blacks, which were nearly double the rates for whites nationwide. Rates for American Indians from 1958 through 1962 were comparable with those of non-Hispanic whites.

Although the age-specific mortality rates for Hispanics and non-Hispanic whites tended to decline from 1958 through 1982 (Figures 3.1 through 3.4) much of the decline was observed between the first and second time periods, 1959 through 62 to 1963 through 67. Age-specific mortality rates for American Indians varied widely, but patterns of change could not be readily interpreted because of the small number of deaths (data not shown).

Colon and Rectum

For this analysis, we combined cancers of the colon and the rectum to minimize the potential for misclassification of primary site, as described

Table 3.3

Cancer mortality rates* in New Mexican females, U.S. white females, and U.S. black females by selected cancer primary sites, 1958 through 1982

Cancer primary site and ethnic group	1958–62	1963–67	1968–72	1973–77	1978–82
Stomach					
NM non-Hispanic white	5.3	3.3	4.2	3.8	3.8
	(61)[a]	(51)	(64)	(67)	(82)
NM Hispanic	17.8	10.5	12.7	9.4	8.9
	(90)	(63)	(76)	(66)	(74)
NM American Indian	6.1	5.8	3.1	4.1	9.4
	(5)	(5)	(3)	(4)	(14)
U.S. white	8.4	6.5	5.1	4.4	3.7
U.S. black	11.6	10.1	7.8	7.1	6.3
Colon and rectum					
NM non-Hispanic white	14.0	12.4	16.8	16.8	14.7
	(159)	(186)	(254)	(294)	(321)
NM Hispanic	9.0	10.9	10.3	12.5	10.9
	(46)	(66)	(63)	(86)	(90)
NM American Indian	3.2	3.9	0.0	5.3	4.6
	(3)	(4)	(0)	(6)	(7)
U.S. white	22.8	21.4	20.7	19.9	18.4
U.S. black	19.2	18.9	20.5	20.6	20.8
Pancreas					
NM non-Hispanic white	4.4	4.6	5.7	6.4	6.3
	(51)	(70)	(87)	(113)	(137)
NM Hispanic	6.1	7.3	6.7	8.3	9.2
	(31)	(44)	(41)	(57)	(76)
NM American Indian	6.8	2.1	6.6	10.1	7.3
	(5)	(2)	(6)	(11)	(10)
U.S. white	6.3	6.6	6.7	6.8	6.8
U.S. black	6.4	7.2	8.3	8.9	9.8
Trachea, bronchus, lung					
NM non-Hispanic white	4.5	6.8	10.8	17.9	19.9
	(53)	(100)	(161)	(305)	(416)
NM Hispanic	4.8	5.3	12.7	12.7	11.2
	(25)	(33)	(76)	(88)	(92)
NM American Indian	1.6	1.9	5.6	2.3	4.2
	(1)	(2)	(5)	(3)	(6)
U.S. white	5.6	7.5	11.1	15.5	21.1
U.S. black	5.7	7.3	11.7	15.4	21.6

Table 3.3 (continued)

Cancer primary site and ethnic group	1958–62	1963–67	1968–72	1973–77	1978–82
Breast					
NM non-Hispanic white	20.3	19.6	24.0	22.1	26.8
	(245)	(287)	(355)	(377)	(559)
NM Hispanic	10.2	11.9	13.3	14.4	19.4
	(63)	(79)	(91)	(109)	(167)
NM American Indian	2.5	4.4	12.6	8.8	8.9
	(3)	(5)	(15)	(11)	(15)
U.S. white	26.2	26.7	27.0	26.9	26.8
U.S. black	23.3	24.3	24.1	25.5	26.6
Cervix uteri					
NM non-Hispanic white	7.0	5.0	4.5	4.0	2.2
	(86)	(73)	(67)	(69)	(45)
NM Hispanic	10.6	9.8	8.1	7.6	4.4
	(66)	(65)	(56)	(56)	(38)
NM American Indian	3.8	9.8	7.8	5.9	7.7
	(4)	(11)	(9)	(8)	(11)
U.S. white	8.1	7.0	5.2	4.0	3.1
U.S. black	19.9	18.0	14.0	11.4	9.0
Corpus and other uterus					
NM non-Hispanic white	4.2	3.0	3.7	3.6	3.8
	(48)	(45)	(56)	(62)	(83)
NM Hispanic	4.6	3.4	4.6	2.9	2.5
	(23)	(21)	(28)	(21)	(21)
NM American Indian	3.4	2.2	0.0	0.0	0.7
	(2)	(2)	(0)	(0)	(1)
U.S. white	6.2	5.3	4.6	4.2	4.0
U.S. black	10.9	9.6	8.1	6.9	7.0
Ovary, Fallopian tube, broad ligament					
NM non-Hispanic white	7.6	6.0	8.3	8.0	7.6
	(91)	(88)	(123)	(136)	(158)
NM Hispanic	5.5	5.7	5.7	7.0	6.2
	(31)	(37)	(38)	(51)	(53)
NM American Indian	8.7	1.4	2.1	2.7	2.2
	(7)	(2)	(2)	(3)	(4)
U.S. white	9.0	9.0	9.1	8.9	8.2
U.S. black	6.8	7.1	7.2	6.7	6.9

Table 3.3 (*continued*)

Cancer primary site and ethnic group	Time period (inclusive years)				
	1958–62	1963–67	1968–72	1973–77	1978–82
Bladder					
NM non-Hispanic white	1.7	1.2	1.7	1.7	1.9
	(19)	(18)	(26)	(31)	(44)
NM Hispanic	1.9	1.9	0.9	1.5	1.3
	(9)	(11)	(5)	(11)	(11)
NM American Indian	0.0	2.1	0.0	0.7	0.0
	(0)	(2)	(0)	(1)	(0)
U.S. white	2.6	2.5	2.3	2.0	2.0
U.S. black	3.7	3.4	3.0	3.0	2.8
Brain					
NM non-Hispanic white	2.8	3.5	2.7	3.4	3.6
	(35)	(49)	(40)	(58)	(72)
NM Hispanic	0.7	2.0	1.8	2.1	1.8
	(7)	(18)	(15)	(19)	(18)
NM American Indian	0.0	0.3	0.0	0.3	0.2
	(0)	(1)	(0)	(1)	(1)
U.S. white	2.8	3.0	3.3	3.5	3.3
U.S. black	1.7	1.6	1.6	1.8	1.9
Hodgkin's lymphoma					
NM non-Hispanic white	1.6	1.0	0.9	0.8	0.4
	(19)	(15)	(14)	(15)	(9)
NM Hispanic	0.2	0.6	1.2	0.9	0.5
	(2)	(6)	(9)	(8)	(5)
NM American Indian	0.0	0.0	0.0	0.0	0.0
	(0)	(0)	(0)	(0)	(0)
U.S. white	1.4	1.4	1.4	0.9	0.7
U.S. black	0.7	0.9	0.7	0.6	0.4
Leukemia					
NM non-Hispanic white	5.6	5.8	5.0	4.8	6.1
	(68)	(81)	(72)	(80)	(126)
NM Hispanic	2.8	4.8	4.4	2.7	4.3
	(22)	(40)	(34)	(23)	(41)
NM American Indian	1.2	0.9	1.8	3.3	1.7
	(2)	(1)	(3)	(6)	(3)
U.S. white[b]	6.0	5.9	5.8	5.3	5.4
U.S. black[b]	4.2	3.9	4.6	4.5	4.7

* Age-adjusted rates per 100,000.
[a] Numbers of deaths are given in parentheses.
[b] Rates for U.S. whites and blacks are calculated for the midpoints of each 5-year interval (1960, 1965, 1970, 1975, 1980).

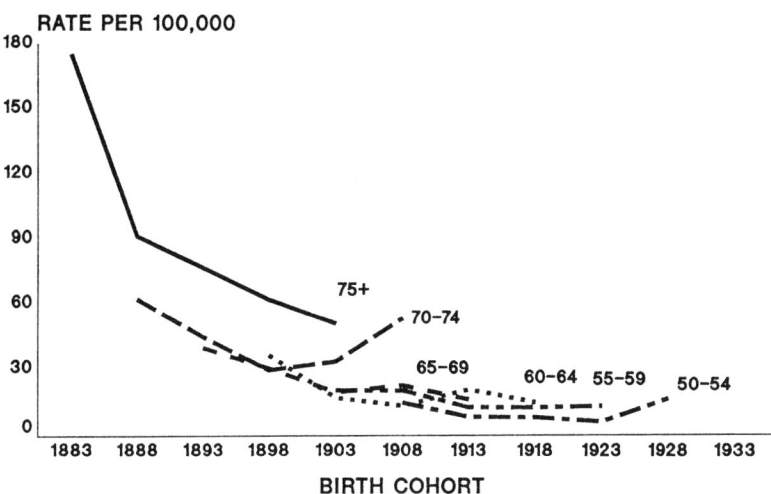

Figure 3.1. *Stomach cancer mortality among non-Hispanic white males in New Mexico, by 5-year birth cohort.*

by Percy, Stanek, and Gloeckler (1981). Colorectal cancer mortality increased among New Mexico males from 1958 through 1982. The increases were more marked among Hispanics and American Indians, with the greatest increases for Hispanic males in the age groups 40 through 44 years, 60 through 64 years, and 75 years and older (Figure 3.5). For non-Hispanic white males, the increments occurred primarily among those 65 years of age and older (Figure 3.6). Colorectal mortality rates were relatively stable for New Mexico females during the period of study (Table 3.3; Figures 3.7 and 3.8). Age-specific mortality rates for American Indians varied widely, and patterns of change of the age-specific rates could not be readily interpreted because of the small number of deaths (data not shown). For both sexes, the risk of death from colorectal cancer was consistently lower for American Indians and Hispanic whites than for non-Hispanic whites.

Pancreas

Pancreatic cancer mortality rates increased during the study period for Hispanic males by 88%, for American Indians by 78%, and for non-

STOMACH CANCER
NON-HISPANIC WHITE FEMALES

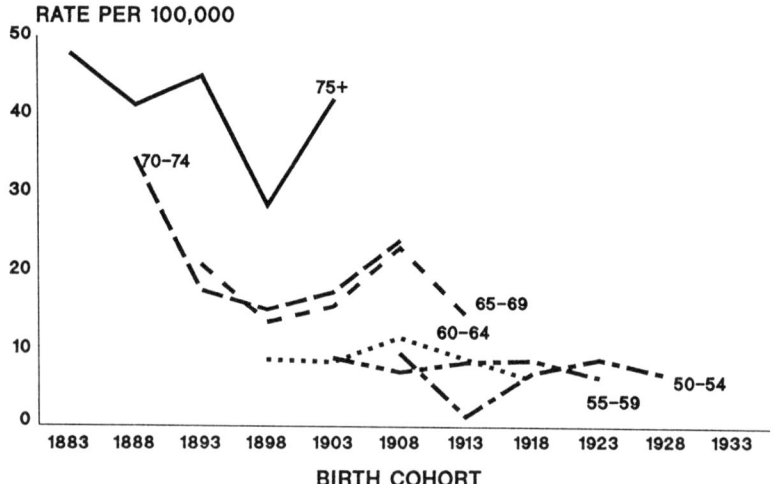

Figure 3.2. *Stomach cancer mortality among non-Hispanic white females in New Mexico, by 5-year birth cohort.*

Hispanic white males by 48% (Table 3.2). Rates also rose for Hispanic and non-Hispanic white females during this period, although the increases were smaller than for males (Table 3.3). The rates for American Indians females varied over the study period but exceeded those of American Indian males in each time period up to 1973 through 1977.

Prostate
Mortality rates for prostate cancer increased in New Mexico during the study period (Table 3.2), rising by 37% for non-Hispanic whites and 74% for Hispanic whites; most of this increase occurred in the latter years of the study period. Mortality rates for American Indians increased by 24% over the same period, but this figure is based on a relatively small number of deaths. Although increases in mortality rates over the period of study were greatest for Hispanics and American Indians, non-Hispanic whites were consistently at highest risk for the disease in New Mexico. Rates for non-Hispanic whites were comparable to those of U.S. whites.

STOMACH CANCER
HISPANIC MALES

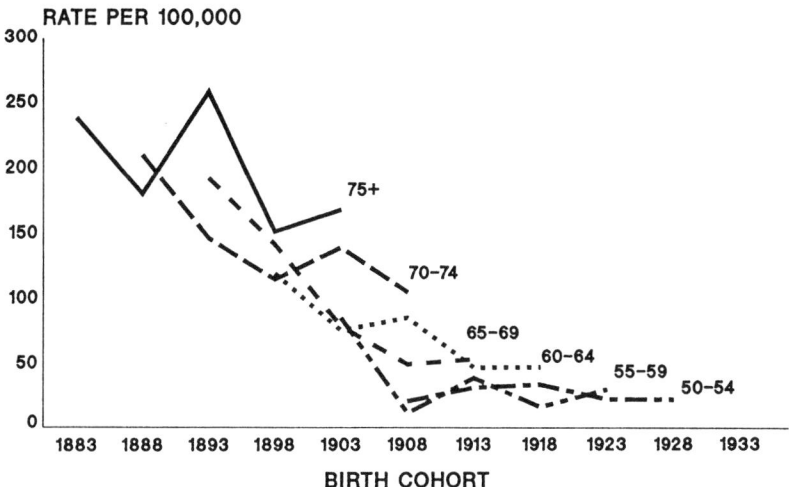

Figure 3.3. *Stomach cancer mortality among Hispanic males in New Mexico, by 5-year birth cohort.*

Bladder
Among males, mortality rates for bladder cancer were highest in non-Hispanic whites, intermediate in Hispanics, and lowest in American Indians. The rates increased across the study period in non-Hispanic and Hispanic whites. The rates were low in females, among whom patterns by ethnic group and time period were not evident.

Female Breast
Breast cancer mortality increased substantially during the period 1958 through 1982 among Hispanic and American Indian women in New Mexico; the rate for non-Hispanic white women also increased, but the increments were less dramatic and less consistent. The greatest increases in Hispanics and non-Hispanic whites were in women aged 50 years and older (Figures 3.9 and 3.10), while in the age groups younger than 50 years, rates were generally stable or declined during the study period. Although the age-adjusted rates for U.S. white women were relatively stable during the study period, the age-specific rates for women 50 years

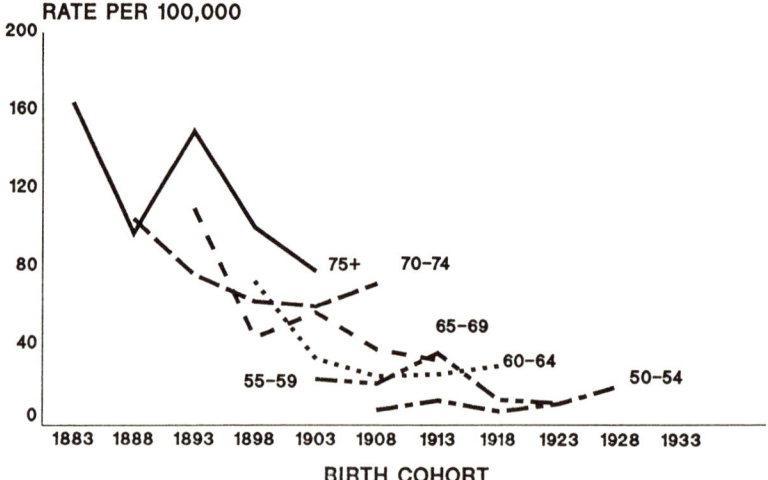

Figure 3.4. *Stomach cancer mortality among Hispanic females in New Mexico, by 5-year birth cohort.*

and older have increased since 1950 (Sondik et al. 1988). Age-specific rates for American Indian females were difficult to interpret because of the small number of deaths. Despite dramatic increases in breast cancer mortality among Hispanics and American Indians, their rates remained well below those of non-Hispanic whites and U.S. whites and blacks.

Cervix uteri
Mortality from cervical cancer in New Mexico declined from 1958 through 1982 (Table 3.3). Mortality rates for non-Hispanic whites were comparable to those for U.S. whites; rates for Hispanics and American Indians were greater than rates for non-Hispanic whites, but generally lower than rates for U.S. blacks. The low mortality rate of 3.8 per 100,000 among American Indian females from 1958 through 1962 increased to 9.8 per 100,000 from 1963 through 1967. We speculate that the low rate during the earlier period followed by a sudden rise in the later period may be the result of a combination of underreporting and the advent of increased screening in the population. However, the appropri-

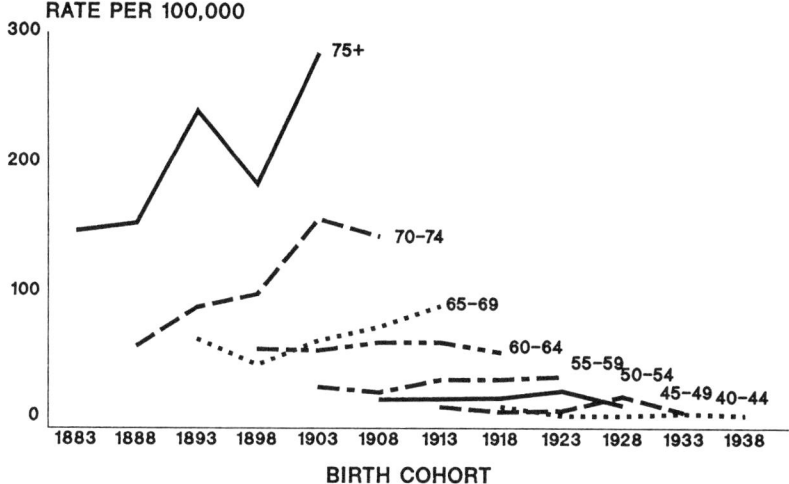

Figure 3.5. *Colorectal cancer mortality among non-Hispanic white males in New Mexico, by 5-year birth cohort.*

ate data for evaluating this hypothesis are not available, and chance variation is also possible.

Corpus and Other Uterus
Mortality rates for uterine cancer declined in the U.S. from 1958 through 1982, though black women remained at higher risk of death from the disease than did whites. Uterine cancer mortality rates were lower among New Mexico women than among U.S. whites and blacks. Rates declined for Hispanic and non-Hispanic white women, but the magnitude of decline was greater among Hispanics than among non-Hispanics. Few deaths from uterine cancer were reported for American Indian women.

Ovary
Mortality rates for cancers of the ovary, Fallopian tube, and broad ligament remained relatively constant from 1958 through 1982, both in New Mexico and in the U.S. New Mexico's non-Hispanic whites were at slightly lower risk of death from these cancers than were U.S. whites, except from 1973 through 1977. Rates for Hispanic women were slightly

36 CHAPTER 3

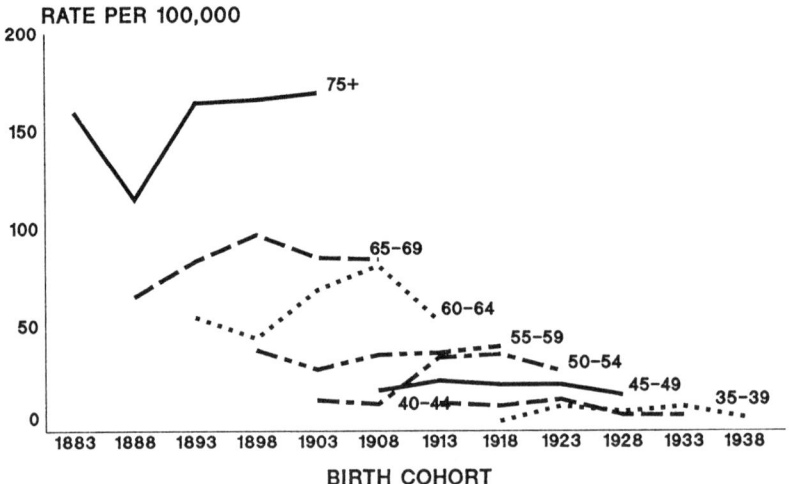

Figure 3.6. *Colorectal cancer mortality among non-Hispanic white females in New Mexico, by 5-year birth cohort.*

lower than those for non-Hispanic whites. Although high rates were observed among American Indian women 1958 through 1962, the rates for subsequent years were much lower than those of Hispanic and non-Hispanic whites.

Brain
Mortality rates for cancers of the brain and nervous system remained relatively stable among U.S. whites and blacks during the study period. Mortality rates for New Mexico non-Hispanic and Hispanic white males increased slightly during the period; comparable rates for females were less variable. The increases in rates were most dramatic for non-Hispanic whites and Hispanic males over the age of 65 years (age-specific data not shown). Rates for American Indians showed no clear pattern of change, and were based on a relatively small number of deaths.

Hodgkin's Lymphoma
Death rates for Hodgkin's lymphoma were lower than for most other cancers presented in this report, and these data may be difficult to inter-

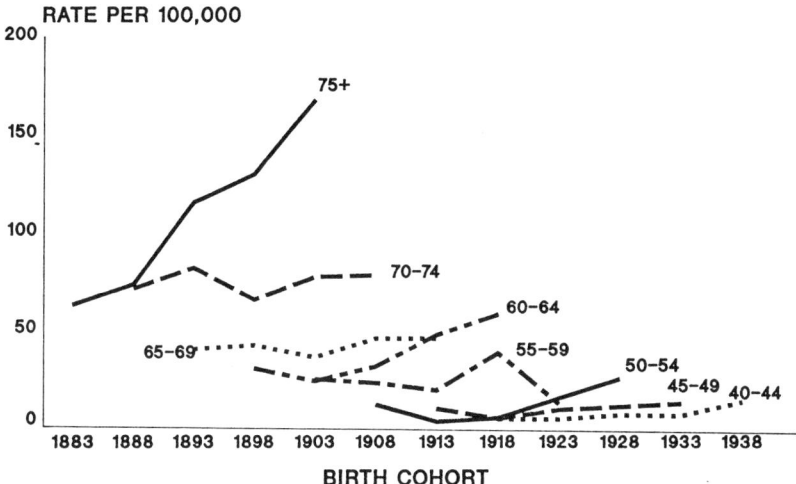

Figure 3.7. *Colorectal cancer mortality among Hispanic males in New Mexico, by 5-year birth cohort.*

pret because of the small number of deaths in this category. Nonetheless, mortality from Hodgkin's lymphoma declined overall for U.S. whites and blacks from 1958 through 1982. Much of the decline occurred in the years after 1973. The mortality experience of New Mexico non-Hispanic whites is similar to that of U.S. whites. Mortality rates for Hispanics varied over the study period and did not show a consistent pattern of decline. Only one death among American Indians was attributed to Hodgkin's lymphoma during the entire period of study.

Leukemia

Mortality rates for leukemia were lower among Hispanics and American Indians than among U.S. whites and New Mexico non-Hispanic whites. Although non-Hispanic white males entered the study period with rates lower than those of U.S. whites, the two groups had similar rates by the final period of the study. Rates for non-Hispanic white females were relatively stable throughout the study. Leukemia mortality rates for U.S. whites and blacks were generally stable during the period, although U.S. black males experienced a slight increase in mortality.

COLORECTAL CANCER MORTALITY
HISPANIC FEMALES

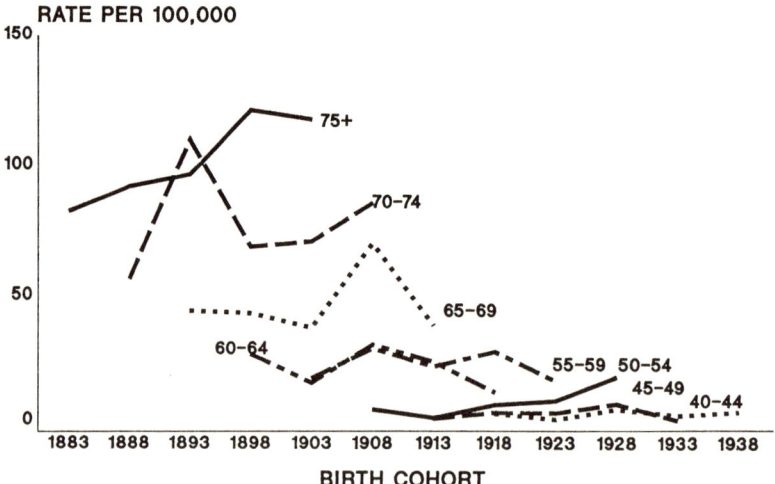

Figure 3.8. *Colorectal cancer mortality among Hispanic females in New Mexico, by 5-year birth cohort.*

Discussion

Our study showed considerable variation in cancer mortality rates by ethnic group and gender in New Mexico during the period 1958 through 1982. Not surprisingly, temporal trends of mortality varied by the primary site of the cancer and, within a given primary site, by ethnic group and gender. While variation in a mortality rate may reflect a true change in the incidence rate of the disease, other factors, including changes in the quality and availability of health care, changes in disease diagnosis and classification, and changes in death certification practices, also affect mortality rates. Rates are also affected by the failure of death certificate information to establish the true primary site of a cancer (Percy, Stanek, and Gloeckler 1981).

In the following sections, we discuss cancer mortality experience in New Mexico in the context of the nationwide experience and in relation to known or suspected etiologic agents for the disease.

Stomach

Stomach cancer mortality rates have declined sharply in many countries during this century (Howson, Hiyama, and Wynder 1986). In the

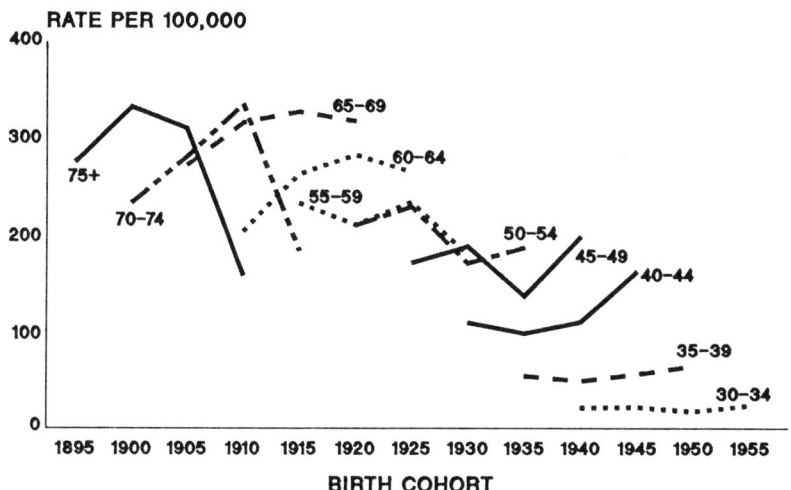

Figure 3.9. *Breast cancer mortality among non-Hispanic white females in New Mexico, by 5-year birth cohort.*

U.S., mortality rates among white males dropped from 37 per 100,000 in 1930 to 9 per 100,000 (70%) in 1977 (Page 1985), and incidence rates dropped 73% from 1950 through 1985 (Sondik et al. 1988). Despite many studies, this downward trend remains unexplained, although changes in diet and in food preparation and storage have been considered as potentially important (Mirvish 1983).

Within the U.S., racial and ethnic differences in the occurrence of stomach cancer are well documented. Incidence and mortality rates for blacks, Japanese, Chinese, and Native Hawaiians are higher than those for whites (Horm et al. 1984). Rates also vary by ethnic group in New Mexico, with American Indians and Hispanics at higher risk than the non-Hispanic white population (Horm et al. 1984).

Among Hispanics in New Mexico, stomach cancer mortality rates declined during the study period, although Hispanics were consistently at greater risk than were non-Hispanic whites. High incidence rates have been reported among other Hispanic populations in the United States (Savitz 1986, Suarez 1980, Menck 1977), in Puerto Rico (Horm et al. 1984), Colombia (Waterhouse et al. 1982), and Spain (Waterhouse et al. 1982). However, data from other locations suggest that both incidence

BREAST CANCER MORTALITY
HISPANIC FEMALES

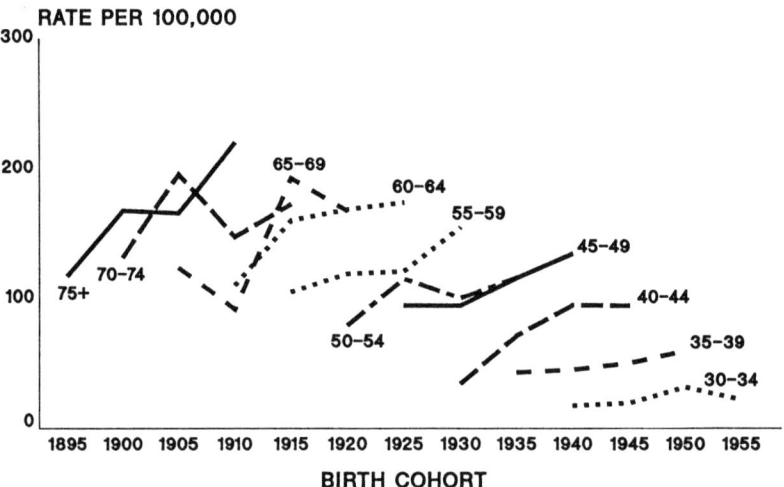

Figure 3.10. *Breast cancer mortality among Hispanic females in New Mexico, by 5-year birth cohort.*

and mortality rates may be declining among Hispanics; for example, Savitz (1986) reported a 42% decline in incidence rates for Spanish-surnamed males in Denver, Colorado, between the periods 1969 through 1971 and 1979 through 1981, although comparable rates for Hispanic females increased slightly. In Texas, a small decline in mortality from stomach cancer was observed among Hispanic males and females between the periods 1968 through 1972 and 1977 through 1980 (Suarez 1980). Nevertheless, rates for Hispanics remained higher than for non-Hispanics in both Colorado and Texas.

Other researchers have found southwestern American Indians to be at lower risk of the disease (Reichenbach 1967, Smith, Salsbury, and Gillian 1956), similar risk (Sievers 1976), and higher risk (Horm *et al.* 1984, Muggia 1971) than are U.S. whites. In New Mexico's American Indians, stomach cancer mortality rates have increased since 1958, and American Indians are now at high risk of disease.

Studies suggest that socioeconomic status is inversely associated with the occurrence of stomach cancer (Howson, Hiyama, and Wynder 1986). In New Mexico, comparisons of census data with stomach cancer incidence and mortality rates are consistent with this observation. The percentage of New Mexico families living below the poverty level in 1979 was 37.9 for American Indians, 20.7 for Hispanics, and 7.1 for non-Hispanic whites (U.S. Bureau of the Census 1981), a pattern that follows the relative ranking of mortality in the three groups in the most recent time period of study (Tables 3.2 and 3.3). The biological correlates of sex, ethnicity, and socioeconomic status in New Mexico that determine stomach cancer risk merit further investigation.

Colon and Rectum

In the U.S., overall mortality rates from cancers of the colon and rectum have declined by approximately 20% since 1950 (Sondik *et al.* 1988), while incidence rates have increased during the same period. The decline in mortality rates in this case probably reflects improvements in diagnostic procedures and treatment.

The etiology of colorectal cancer is poorly understood. The present hypotheses emphasize the role of diet, particularly fat and fiber intake (Modan 1977). Families at high risk for colon cancer have been well documented, suggesting a genetic component for some cancers of this site (Kussin, Lipkin, and Winawer 1979).

The distribution of dietary factors related to the etiology of colorectal cancer is not well defined in New Mexico. However, recent increases in the disease among Hispanics and American Indians suggest that changes in diet that accompany acculturation to the non-Hispanic white lifestyle could be a factor.

Pancreas

In New Mexico, pancreatic cancer mortality rates rose during the study period for all groups except American Indian females, whose rates were, however, consistently higher than rates for American Indian males.

Temporal and ethnic patterns of pancreatic cancer mortality are difficult to interpret, and it is not possible to determine from our results whether the increased rates represent a true rise in the incidence of the disease. Increased rates could be the result of inconsistent vital record certification and changes in diagnostic procedures, and of greater access to health care, a factor that varies by ethnicity and socioeconomic status in most locations.

Risk factors for pancreatic cancer include cigarette smoking, diabetes mellitus, alcohol consumption, and chronic pancreatitis (Mack 1982). The smoking habits of New Mexico's non-Hispanic whites are similar to those of whites nationwide, while Hispanics and American Indians generally consume less tobacco than do non-Hispanic whites (Samet *et al.*

1982; Samet *et al.* 1988a). Although a recent study suggests an increase in tobacco consumption among young Hispanics (Greenberg *et al.* 1987), cigarette smoking would probably not have been an important cause of pancreatic cancer among Hispanics and American Indians during the period of the present study. Hispanics and American Indians are at high risk for diabetes mellitus (Samet 1988b; Gohdes 1986; West 1978), and a high prevalence of alcohol abuse has been reported in these populations (May 1986). However, the relative contribution of these factors to pancreatic cancer in Hispanics and American Indians remains unknown.

Prostate
Nationwide, incidence rates for prostate cancer increased by 67% among white males from 1947 through 1984 (Devesa *et al.* 1987). In contrast, the corresponding mortality rates remained relatively constant. Before 1945, the rates for prostate cancer were higher for whites than for blacks. However, dramatic increases in the incidence of, and mortality from, the disease among U.S. blacks have since placed them at greater risk than U.S. whites for the disease.

Survival after the diagnosis of prostate cancer has improved since the 1950's, and the improvement may partially explain the relatively constant mortality rates despite increases in incidence. Improved treatment modalities may be partially responsible for better survival, especially for patients with advanced disease. However, improved diagnostic techniques may provide for earlier diagnosis and more accurate staging of the disease. Because a large proportion of elderly men have asymptomatic prostate cancer (Greenwald 1982), improved diagnostic techniques may have identified less aggressive forms of the disease that would not previously have been diagnosed. Further, earlier diagnosis of prostate tumors could result in apparently improved survival as the result of "lead time" bias.

Despite extensive study, the causes of prostate cancer are unknown. Although the disease may involve a genetic mechanism, much of the evidence to date is consistent with an environmental etiology. Diet, sexual practices, and hormonal factors have all been implicated in the etiology of the disease (Greenwald 1982). Excess occurrence of prostate cancer has been associated with occupational exposures to cadmium (Kolonel and Winkelstein 1977) and has been observed among rubber workers (Tyroler *et al.* 1976). The differences observed in prostate cancer mortality rates among non-Hispanic whites, Hispanics, and American Indians cannot be readily explained. The rates tend to be lowest in American Indians and lower in Hispanics than in non-Hispanic whites. However, the magnitude of these differences is not large.

Bladder

Cigarette smoking and certain occupational agents have been causally linked to cancer of the bladder (International Agency for Research on Cancer 1986). The observed pattern in New Mexico, with the highest rates in non-Hispanic white males, is consistent with differences in cigarette-smoking practices among the ethnic groups in the state. However, occupational exposures sustained outside New Mexico might contribute to the elevated rates in non-Hispanic white males.

Female Breast

Risk factors for breast cancer include socioeconomic status, age at menarche, age at first birth of a child, parity, radiation, the presence of fibrocystic disease, family history, and, possibly, diet (Petrakis, Ernster, and King 1982). Studies that have correlated the occurrence of breast cancer with socioeconomic status have found that the highest rates occur in the upper socioeconomic status levels. Ecological comparisons of census data with breast cancer mortality rates for New Mexico are consistent with these observations: non-Hispanic whites generally have a higher socioeconomic status level than do Hispanics, who in turn generally have a higher education and economic level than do American Indians (U.S. Bureau of the Census 1981). This pattern is consistent with the relative ranking of breast cancer mortality during the period of study.

Nulliparity and increased age (>30 years) at first pregnancy have been associated with increased risk of breast cancer. High rates of fertility in New Mexico's Hispanic and American Indian populations may contribute to the low risk of breast cancer in these populations relative to non-Hispanic whites. On average, age at first pregnancy is probably lower in the American Indians and Hispanics, although we are not aware of specific data to support this speculation. However, high dietary fat and obesity may also be associated with increased risk. Hispanics (Samet et al. 1988b) and American Indians (West 1978) are at high risk for obesity, and the low rates of breast cancer in these groups are not consistent with the latter hypothesis. Mortality rates increased in Hispanic women during the period 1958 through 1982. Data from the New Mexico Tumor Registry document a rising incidence from the 1970's through the 1980's. We lack the needed longitudinal data on risk factors to explain the temporal trend of increasing breast cancer mortality.

Cervix Uteri

The development of the Papanicolaou smear technique in the 1940's offered a technique for decreasing morbidity and mortality from cervical cancer (Cramer 1982). Declining incidence and mortality rates from cervical cancer during the latter half of this century are probably the result of the widespread implementation of the Pap smear (Guzick 1978). In the United States, mortality from invasive cervical cancer declined steadily from 1958 through 1982 (Devesa *et al.* 1987). Although temporal patterns among blacks for this disease were similar to nationwide trends, U.S. blacks remained at higher risk of death from cervical cancer than did U.S. whites throughout the study period.

Factors that increase the risk for cervical cancer include an early age at first intercourse, a high number of sexual partners, vaginal deliveries of babies, low socioeconomic status, exposure to sexually transmitted diseases, and, possibly, low dietary vitamin A, C, and folate intake (Cramer 1982). However, age at first intercourse and number of sexual partners have emerged as two of the stronger risk factors for the disease. The increased risk of cervical cancer associated with the number of sexual partners is probably related to the increased chances of contracting a sexually transmitted disease (Cramer 1982). Sexually transmitted diseases have been implicated in the genesis of cervical cancer; human papillomavirus, a sexually transmitted infection, is currently receiving widespread attention as a possible etiologic agent of the disease (Peto and zur Hausen 1986).

The distribution of these risk factors in cervical cancer cases in New Mexico is not known. However, preliminary data from ongoing studies of preinvasive cervical lesions (dysplasia) in New Mexico indicate that Hispanic and American Indian women with cervical dysplasia give histories of few lifetime sex partners and few episodes of sexually transmitted diseases (Buckley 1991). In addition, laboratory data collected on women with cervical dysplasia in all three major ethnic groups in the state show few positive cervical culture results for sexually transmitted microbiologic organisms. It is possible that the epidemiology of cervical disease in New Mexico may differ from that reported in other populations.

Corpus and Other Uterus
Obesity and the use of exogenous estrogens are the two risk factors most commonly associated with cancer of the uterus. Although Hispanic women tend to be more obese than non-Hispanic white women, rates are comparable in the two groups (Samet *et al.* 1988b). Data are not available on estrogen use for women in New Mexico.

The endometrium is one of the few cancer sites for which some studies have shown an inverse relationship with cigarette smoking; that is, smoking is associated with a lower risk of the disease. The low prevalence of cigarette smoking among Hispanics and American Indians (Samet *et al.*

1988a) might be expected to increase mortality from endometrial cancer, but a consistent pattern is not evident on review of Table 3.3.

Ovary

Age-adjusted mortality rates for cancer of the ovary remained relatively constant in the U.S. from 1950 through 1980 (Sondik *et al.* 1988). However, masked in the stability of the age-adjusted rates were increases in rates among women over 50 years of age and declining rates in women under 50. New Mexico non-Hispanic white females show similar patterns (age-specific data not shown). Age-specific rates for Hispanics and American Indian females are more variable, mostly because of the small number of deaths from this disease in the two groups. Nonetheless, the net effect of changes in age-specific mortality is that age-adjusted ovarian cancer mortality rates in New Mexico, as in the U.S., changed little during the period of this study.

The etiology of ovarian tumors remains unclear, though estrogens seem to mediate the development of the disease. Having children is associated with a lower risk of disease, as is consumption of exogenous estrogens (Weiss 1982). In New Mexico, fertility rates of Hispanics and American Indians are higher than those of non-Hispanic whites (State of New Mexico 1990), and are consistent with the lower risk of ovarian cancer among those groups. Estrogen use in the three ethnic populations is not well characterized in New Mexico. Other potential etiologic agents include radiation, talc, and asbestos (Weiss 1982), but exposure to these factors has not been assessed in New Mexico women.

Brain

Increased rates of mortality from brain cancer were observed among U.S. whites, aged 65 through 84 years, during the period 1968 through 83 (Davis and Schwartz 1988). Rates for New Mexico Hispanic males and non-Hispanic whites of both sexes were consistent with this trend. Rates for Hispanic females and American Indians were variable and based on a small number of deaths.

The increased rates of brain cancer mortality may be the result of better diagnostic capabilities and subsequent improvements in the reporting of vital data. However, some investigators believe that the observed increases cannot be fully explained by improvements in diagnostic techniques (Davis and Schwartz 1988).

Hodgkin's Lymphoma

Deaths from Hodgkin's lymphoma are rare in the U.S. and in New Mexico. Rates for New Mexico's Hispanics and non-Hispanic whites were based on a small number of deaths, and showed little variation during the study period. It is remarkable that only one death from Hodgkin's disease was recorded among American Indians in New Mexico during the entire period of this study. Problems with death certification may partially explain this observation, however, incidence data from the New Mexico Tumor Registry also suggest that cases of Hodgkin's lymphoma are rare among southwestern American Indians (Duncan et al. 1986; Horm et al. 1984).

Leukemia
In the U.S., incidence rates of leukemia increased from 1950 through 1975, then declined through 1985 (Devesa et al. 1987). During this period, leukemia mortality rates increased only slightly, reflecting marked improvements in survival from this group of hematopoietic diseases (Sondik et al. 1988). The temporal trends in mortality rates in New Mexico are consistent with the nationwide experience. However, rates among Hispanics and American Indians remained well below those of non-Hispanic whites and U.S. whites during the study period.

Environmental risk factors for leukemia include exposure to ionizing radiation, benzene, and certain alkylating agents used in chemotherapy (Heath 1982). Genetic factors and viral infections may also play a role in the etiology of the leukemias (Heath 1982). There is mounting evidence of an association between nonionizing radiation and the development of leukemia, though this remains controversial (Savitz, Pearce, and Poole 1989). As with most cancers, the distribution of risk factors for leukemia has not been adequately studied in New Mexico.

Summary

With a few notable exceptions, cancer mortality rates for New Mexico's non-Hispanic whites were similar to those of U.S. whites, while Hispanics and American Indians were generally at lower risk of death from cancer. Stomach cancer mortality rates in New Mexico Hispanics and non-Hispanic whites followed the decline observed worldwide. Nonetheless, Hispanics and American Indians remained at higher risk of death from stomach cancer than did non-Hispanic whites. Colorectal cancer mortality rates increased among New Mexico males, most notably in Hispanics and American Indians, and remained stable for New Mexico females. Mortality rates for cancers of the pancreas, prostate, and breast also increased during the study period, while rates for cervical cancer and uterine cancer declined. Mortality rates for Hodgkin's disease were lower in

New Mexico than in the U.S., with an almost complete lack of the disease observed among American Indians.

The descriptive epidemiology of cancer in New Mexico is well documented (Horm *et al.* 1984, Key and Lerchen 1987). However, except for cancers of cigarette-related sites, we lack the data needed to explain the patterns of racial and ethnic variation. The New Mexico Tumor Registry will continue to serve as an important resource for monitoring changes in cancer incidence among the state's Hispanics, American Indians, and non-Hispanic whites. The Registry also provides a base for future cohort and case-control studies that may help to clarify the reasons for the differing patterns of cancer occurrence in New Mexico's diverse population.

REFERENCES

Buckley, D. I., R. S. McPherson, C. Q. North, and T. M. Becker. 1991. Dietary micronutrients and cervical dysplasia in southwestern American Indian women. Abstract. *Clinical Research* 39:76A.

Cramer, D. W. 1982. Uterine cervix. In *Cancer epidemiology and prevention,* edited by D. Schottenfeld and J. F. Fraumeni, Jr., 881–900. Philadelphia: Saunders.

Davis, D. L., and J. Schwartz. 1988. Trends in cancer mortality: U.S. white males and females, 1968–83. *Lancet* 1:633–636.

Devesa, S. S., D. T. Silverman, J. L. Young, Jr., *et al.* 1987. Cancer incidence and mortality trends among whites in the United States, 1947–84. *J.Natl.Cancer Inst.* 79:701–770.

Duncan, M. H., C. L. Wiggins, C. R. Key, and J. M. Samet. 1986. Childhood cancer epidemiology in New Mexico's American Indians, Hispanic whites, and non-Hispanic whites, 1970–82. *J.Natl.Cancer Inst.* 76:1013–1018.

Gohdes, D. M. 1986. Diabetes in American Indians: a growing problem. *Diabetes Care* 9:609–613.

Greenberg, M. A., C. L. Wiggins, D. M. Kutvirt, and J. M. Samet. 1987. Cigarette use among Hispanic and non-Hispanic white school children, Albuquerque, New Mexico. *Am.J.Public Health* 77:621–622.

Greenwald, P. 1982. Prostate. In *Cancer epidemiology and prevention,* edited by D. Schottenfeld and J. F. Fraumeni, Jr., 938–946. Philadelphia: Saunders.

Guzick, D. S. 1978. Efficacy of screening for cervical cancer: a review. *Am.J. Public Health* 68:125–134.

Heath, C. W., Jr. 1982. The leukemias. In *Cancer epidemiology and prevention,* edited by D. Schottenfeld and J. F. Fraumeni, Jr., 728–738. Philadelphia: Saunders.

Horm, J. W., A. J. Asire, J. L. Young, Jr., and E. S. Pollack 1984. *SEER Program: cancer incidence and mortality in the United States 1973–1981.* NIH publication No. 85–1837. Bethesda, MD: National Cancer Institute.

Howson, C. P., T. Hiyama, and E. L. Wynder. 1986. The decline in gastric cancer: epidemiology of an unplanned triumph. *Epidemiol.Rev.* 8:1–27.

International Agency for Research on Cancer. 1986. *IARC monographs on the evaluation of the carcinogenic risk of chemicals to humans: tobacco smoking.* Vol. 38. Lyon, France.

Key, C. R. and M. Lerchen. 1987. USA: New Mexico. In *Cancer incidence in five continents,* edited by C. Muir, J. Waterhouse, T. Mack., J. Powell, and S. Whelan, Vol. V. IARC Scientific Publication No. 88. International Agency for Research on Cancer. Lyon, France.

Kolonel, L., and W. Winkelstein, Jr. 1977. Cadmium and prostatic carcinoma. *Lancet* 2:566–567.

Kussin, S. Z., M. Lipkin, and S. J. Winawer. 1979. Inherited colon cancer: clinical implications. *Am.J.Gastroenterol.* 72:448–457.

Mack, T. M. 1982. Pancreas. In *Cancer epidemiology and prevention,* edited by D. Schottenfeld and J. F. Fraumeni, Jr., 638–667. Philadelphia: Saunders.

May, P. A. 1986. Alcohol and drug misuse prevention programs for American Indians: needs and opportunities. *J.Stud.Alcohol* 47:187–195.

Menck, H. R. 1977. Cancer incidence in the Mexican American. *Natl.Cancer Inst.Monogr.* 47:103–106.

Mirvish, S. S. 1983. The etiology of gastric cancer. Intragastric nitrosamide formation and other theories. *J.Natl.Cancer Inst.* 71:629–647.

Modan, B. 1977. Role of diet in cancer etiology. *Cancer* 40:1887–1891.

Muggia, A. L. 1971. Diseases among the Navajo Indians. *Rocky Mt.Med.J.* 68:39–49.

Page, H. S., and A. J. Asire. 1985. *Cancer rates and risks.* NIH Publication No. 85–691. Bethesda, MD: National Cancer Institute.

Percy, C., E. Stanek III, and L. Gloeckler. 1981. Accuracy of cancer death certificates and its effect on cancer mortality statistics. *Am.J.Public Health* 71:242–250.

Peto, R. and H. zur Hausen. 1986. *Viral etiology of cervical cancer.* Branbury Report 21. Cold Spring Harbor, NY: Cold Spring Harbor Laboratory.

Petrakis, N. L., V. L. Ernster, and M. C. King. 1982. Breast. In *Cancer epidemiology and prevention,* edited by D. Schottenfeld and J. F. Fraumeni, Jr., 855–870. Philadelphia: Saunders.

Reichenbach, D. D. 1967. Autopsy incidence of diseases among Southwestern American Indians. *Arch.Pathol.* 84:81–86.

Samet, J. M., S. D. Schrag, C. A. Howard, C. R. Key, and D. R. Pathak. 1982. Respiratory disease in a New Mexico population sample of Hispanic and non-Hispanic whites. *Am.Rev.Respir.Dis.* 125:152–157.

Samet, J. M., C. L. Wiggins, C. R. Key, and T. M. Becker. 1988a. Mortality from lung cancer and chronic obstructive pulmonary disease in New Mexico, 1958–82. *Am.J.Public Health* 78:1182–1186.

Samet, J. M., D. B. Coultas, C. A. Howard, *et al.* 1988b. Diabetes, gallbladder disease, obesity, and hypertension among Hispanics in New Mexico. *Am.J. Epidemiol.* 128:1302–1311.

Savitz, D. A. 1986. Changes in Spanish surname cancer rates relative to other whites, Denver area, 1969–71 to 1979–81. *Am.J.Public Health* 76:1210–1215.

Savitz, D. A., N. E. Pearce, and C. Poole. 1989. Methodological issues in the epidemiology of electromagnetic fields and cancer. *Epidemiol.Rev.* 11:59–78.

Sievers, M. L. 1976. Cancer of the digestive system among American Indians. *Ariz.Med.* 33:15–20.

Smith, R. L., C. G. Salsbury, and A. G. Gilliam. 1956. Recorded and expected mortality among the Navajo, with special reference to cancer. *J.Natl.Cancer Inst.* 17:77–89.

Sondik, E., J. Young, Jr., J. Horm, and L. Gloeckler-Ries. 1988. *Annual cancer statistics review including cancer trends: 1950–1985.* Bethesda, MD: National Cancer Institute.

Suarez, L., and J. Martin. 1987. Epidemiology of cancer mortality in Texas, 1969–1980. Austin, Texas: Texas Department of Health.

State of New Mexico, Health and Environment Department, Public Health Division, Vital Records and Statistics. May 1990. *New Mexico selected health statistics 1988 annual report.*

Tyroler, H. A., D. Andjelkovic, R. Harris, *et al.* 1976. Chronic disease in the rubber industry. *Environ.Health Perspect.* 17:13–20.

U.S. Bureau of the Census. 1981. *Census of the population, 1980. General social and economic characteristics: New Mexico.* Final Report PC80-1-C33. Washington, DC: U.S. Government Printing Office.

Waterhouse, J., C. Muir, K. Shanmugaratnam, and J. Powell, eds. 1982. *Cancer incidence in five continents.* IARC Scientific Publication No. 42, Vol. 4. Lyon, France: International Agency for Research on Cancer.

Weiss, N. S. 1982. Ovary. In *Cancer epidemiology and prevention,* edited by D. Schottenfeld and J. R. Fraumeni, Jr., 871–880. 1982. Philadelphia: Saunders.

West, K. M. 1978. Diabetes in American Indians. *Adv.Metab.Dis.* 9:29.

CHAPTER 4

Diabetes Mortality

Janette S. Carter
Charles L. Wiggins
Thomas M. Becker
Charles R. Key
Jonathan M. Samet

Diabetes is an important cause of morbidity and mortality in the U.S. In 1985, diabetes was the seventh leading cause of death in the U.S., and the thirteenth leading cause of years of potential life lost (YPLL) before age 65 years (Centers for Disease Control 1988). Mortality rates from diabetes reflect diverse factors that include the prevalence of disease, patterns of death certification, and the case-fatality ratio. The case-fatality ratio may be influenced by both the clinical characteristics of the disease and access to care and self-care practices.

Diabetes mortality rates in the U.S. vary among racial and ethnic groups; blacks, for example, have higher death rates nationwide than do whites in all age groups (Harris and Entmacher 1985); and in Bexar County, Texas, Spanish-surname residents have rates two to four times higher than do non-Spanish-surname residents (Stern and Gaskill 1978). The variation in diabetes mortality rates among various ethnic populations parallels differences in diabetes prevalence rates. Blacks (Roseman 1985), American Indians (Bennett and Knowler 1979; Gohdes 1986), and Hispanics (Diehl and Stern 1989; Hamman *et al.* 1989; Perez-Stable *et al.* 1989) all show higher prevalence figures than do whites nationwide. Studies also show that Hispanics, compared with whites nationwide, may have more severe disease, as manifested by the higher prevalence of diabetes complications (Haffner, Fong, and Stern 1988; Pugh *et al.* 1988) and by the larger proportion of Hispanics receiving pharmacologic treatments for the disease (Haffner *et al.* 1984).

The prevalence of diabetes among Hispanic (Samet *et al.* 1988) and American Indian (Carter *et al.* 1989) populations in New Mexico is high, but the diabetes-related mortality rates for these two groups have not been compared with the mortality rates for non-Hispanic whites in the state. To this end, we analyzed vital record data to examine differences in diabetes-related mortality in New Mexico's Hispanic, American Indian, and non-Hispanic white populations, and to determine whether temporal trends in mortality in these populations followed nationwide trends.

Methodologic Considerations

Cause of death was coded according to the seventh revision of the International Classification of Diseases (ICD) for the years 1958 through 1968 (World Health Organization [WHO] 1957), the eighth ICD revision for the years 1969 through 1978 (WHO 1967), and the ninth ICD revision for the years 1979 through 1982 (WHO 1977). For this report, deaths attributed to diabetes included ICD 260 in the seventh revision and ICD 250 in the eighth and ninth revisions. Because the comparability ratios between the seventh and eighth ICD revisions were 0.9971 (National Center for Health Statistics [NCHS] 1975a) and 0.9991 (NCHS 1980a), respectively, we did not make any adjustments for the different ICD revisions. Census figures for the diabetes mortality rates in the U.S. white population for the 25-year period were obtained from published sources for comparison (NCHS 1960, 1965, 1970, 1975b 1980b).

Results

The age-adjusted diabetes mortality rates for males and for females in the three major ethnic groups in New Mexico are shown in Tables 4.1 and 4.2; U.S. white rates (NCHS 1960, 1965, 1970, 1975b, 1980b) are included for comparison. Substantial differences were observed among ethnic groups, with rates for Hispanics and American Indians exceeding rates for non-Hispanic whites in most of the time periods analyzed. During the last 5-year period, the highest age-adjusted mortality rates were among Hispanic males and American Indian females.

A marked increase was apparent in the age-adjusted mortality rates for Hispanics and American Indians during the 25-year period. The rates for American Indian females, which began as the lowest of any group, increased nearly 400% through the last 5-year period. The rates for American Indian males increased by 93%. Rates for Hispanic males and females also rose sharply. Mortality rates for non-Hispanic whites in New Mexico also increased over the 25-year period but were less dramatic, with an increase of 50% for males and 11% for females. The increase in

Table 4.1
Diabetes mortality rates* in New Mexican males and U.S. white males, 1958 through 1982

	Time period (inclusive years)				
	1958–62	1963–67	1968–72	1973–77	1978–82
Non-Hispanic white	12.0	13.3	13.4	12.2	18.0
	(118)[a]	(157)	(156)	(166)	(293)
Hispanic	10.5	16.0	23.0	21.8	27.9
	(55)	(92)	(136)	(143)	(203)
American Indian	11.6	10.5	26.2	24.9	22.4
	(10)	(10)	(28)	(30)	(29)
U.S. white	15.3	15.8	17.1	14.6	13.0

* Age-adjusted rates per 100,000.
[a] Numbers of deaths are given in parentheses.

Table 4.2
Diabetes mortality rates* in New Mexican females and U.S. white females, 1958 through 1982

	Time period (inclusive years)				
	1958–62	1963–67	1968–72	1973–77	1978–82
Non-Hispanic white	13.5	9.6	12.0	12.3	15.0
	(154)[a]	(145)	(184)	(216)	(329)
Hispanic	15.7	19.8	27.3	24.5	28.6
	(84)	(120)	(167)	(170)	(234)
American Indian	6.6	7.7	26.0	18.0	32.2
	(5)	(7)	(26)	(20)	(46)
U.S. white	18.5	17.6	17.8	14.4	12.3

* Age-adjusted rates per 100,000.
[a] Numbers of deaths are given in parentheses.

rates for New Mexico whites contrasted with a decrease in rates for U.S. whites during the latter part of the 25-year period.

Figures 4.1 through 4.4 show the age-specific diabetes mortality rates for successive birth cohorts for Hispanics and non-Hispanic whites. Figures for American Indians are not included because of the small numbers of deaths for each age group. Overall, higher mortality rates were observed for Hispanics than for non-Hispanic whites. The rates increased in the older age groups for both Hispanics and non-Hispanic whites, but more steeply for Hispanics. Although the numbers of deaths were small in

DIABETES
NON-HISPANIC WHITE MALES

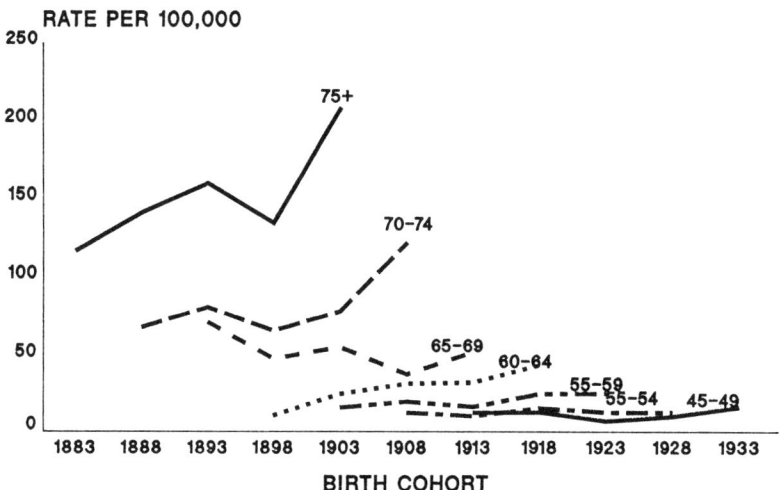

Figure 4.1. *Diabetes mortality among non-Hispanic white males in New Mexico, by 5-year birth cohort.*

the younger age groups, Hispanics appeared to have higher mortality rates than did non-Hispanic whites.

Discussion

Our analysis of diabetes-related mortality rates from 1958 through 1982 reveals substantial differences among New Mexico's three major ethnic groups, with American Indians and Hispanics having the highest rates. A marked increase was apparent in the age-adjusted mortality rates for Hispanics and American Indians, with a smaller increase for non-Hispanic whites during the 25-year period. This pattern of continually increasing diabetes mortality rates contrasts with the rates for U.S. whites, which peaked in the 5-year period 1968 through 1972 and then declined. The differences in mortality rates among the three major ethnic groups in New Mexico reflect the multiple factors that determine diabetes mortality (Figure 4.5).

The prevalence of diabetes and its complications can be measured, but

DIABETES
NON-HISPANIC WHITE FEMALES

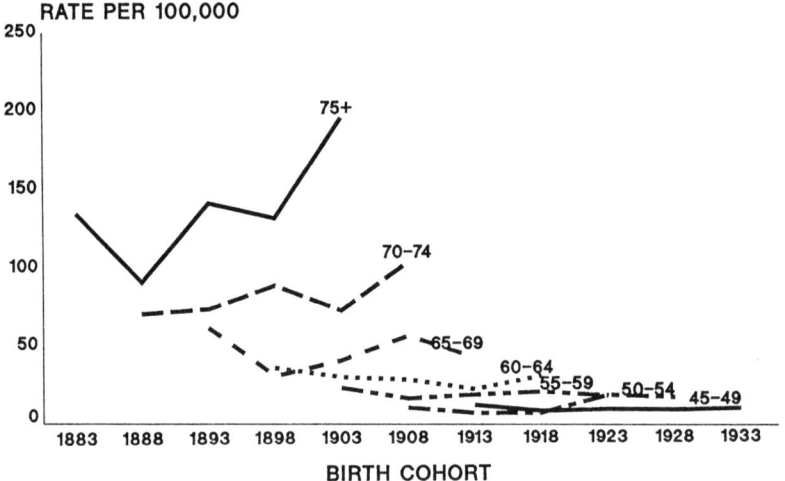

Figure 4.2. *Diabetes mortality among non-Hispanic white females in New Mexico, by 5-year birth cohort.*

it is difficult to assess the impact of health care delivery and patient behavior on diabetes mortality. Some impediments to care extend across cultural and ethnic boundaries; for example, the rural nature of the State of New Mexico and the low socioeconomic status of many of its citizens (New Mexico Health and Environment Department 1988). Other impediments exist within cultural groups; for example, the unique social systems and health beliefs of Hispanics and American Indians may create barriers to care that differ from those faced by non-Hispanic whites, and may affect the risk of death from diabetes.

In addition, deaths of persons with diabetes may be coded differently in New Mexico than in other states, and within the state, coding may vary among the ethnic groups because of different competing causes of death. For example, ischemic heart disease, an important cause of death in persons with diabetes, is associated with the highest mortality rates for non-Hispanic whites, intermediate rates for Hispanics, and the lowest rates for American Indians (Becker *et al.* 1988). This pattern of mortality might increase the diabetes mortality rate for American Indians and Hispanics relative to the rate for non-Hispanic whites. Lastly, coding for

DIABETES
HISPANIC MALES

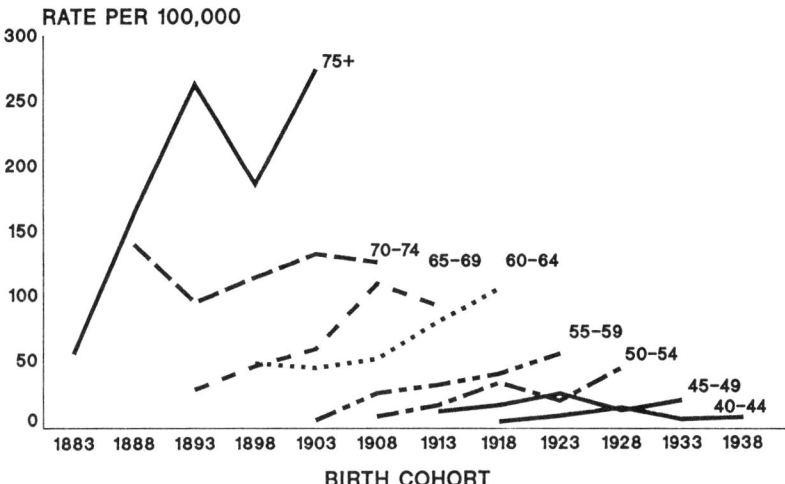

Figure 4.3. *Diabetes mortality among Hispanic males in New Mexico, by 5-year birth cohort.*

diabetes could differ in New Mexico from coding used nationwide. If patients with diabetes are not receiving consistent medical care, it is less likely that a diagnosis of diabetes will be noted at the time of death and later coded on the death certificate. Factors affecting diabetes mortality rates for each ethnic group are discussed below.

Non-Hispanic Whites
The prevalence and complications of diabetes among the non-Hispanic white population of New Mexico have not been investigated; however, many indicators point to a lower status of health care in the state as compared with health care nationwide (New Mexico Health and Environment Department 1988). New Mexico is consistently ranked in the bottom 10 states in per capita income, and approximately 25% of the population has no third-party coverage for health services, as compared to 15% of the U.S. population. New Mexico ranks 44th among the states in per capita personal health care expenditures, and 29 of the state's 33 counties had some portion of the county designated as a health manpower shortage area in 1987. Geographic isolation is apparent in the

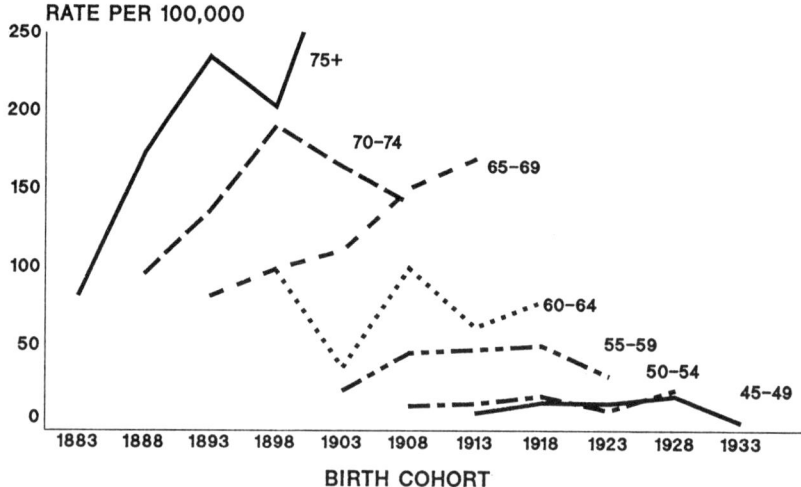

Figure 4.4. *Diabetes mortality among Hispanic females in New Mexico, by 5-year birth cohort.*

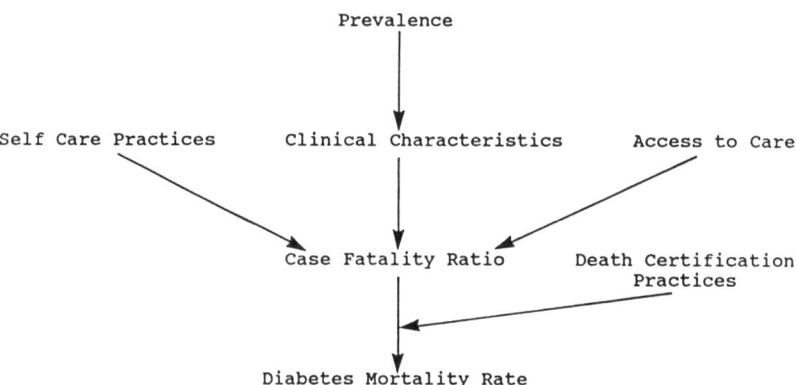

Figure 4.5. *Multiple factors that affect the diabetes mortality rate.*

state, with 17 counties having a population density of fewer than 6 per square mile, 14 counties having 6 to 100 per square mile, and only two counties with more than 100 per square mile.

In the rural areas of the state, it is likely that many patients have a long duration of symptoms before diagnosis and treatment, a factor that was found to be one of five contributing to a predictive index for death in a British study. Close professional surveillance and significant patient participation are required for optimal diabetes care, but neither of these can be achieved in a setting of limited health care access because of financial and geographic constraints. In fact, the continued rise of diabetes mortality among non-Hispanic whites in the state corresponds to similar patterns seen in developing countries.

Hispanics

Diabetes is more common, and may also be more severe, in Hispanics as compared with non-Hispanic whites. In the U.S. (Perez-Stable *et al.* 1989) and in the Southwest (Diehl and Stern 1989; Hamman *et al.* 1989), the prevalence of diabetes among Hispanics is at least twice that among non-Hispanic whites. Data for New Mexico also show a high prevalence of diabetes in Hispanics (Samet *et al.* 1988; New Mexico Health and Environment Department 1987). The high prevalence of diabetes in Hispanics would be expected to cause a proportional increase in Hispanic mortality ratios compared with non-Hispanic white rates, assuming a case-fatality rate in Hispanics at least equal to that in non-Hispanic whites.

The San Antonio Heart Study demonstrates differences in the clinical characteristics of diabetes between Hispanic and non-Hispanic whites. In comparison with non-Hispanic whites, Hispanics have an earlier age at onset of diabetes, higher 1-hour postprandial serum glucose, larger proportions receiving pharmacologic treatments for diabetes (Haffner *et al.* 1984), and increased risk of severe diabetic retinopathy (Haffner, Fong, and Stern 1988) and diabetic end-stage renal disease (Pugh *et al.* 1988). In contrast, however, preliminary information from the San Luis Valley diabetes study did not show ethnic group differences in Colorado (Hamman *et al.* 1988). In New Mexico, Hispanics have a genetic background similar to that of the Hispanic people of the San Luis Valley, so we might expect similar clinical characteristics (Nostrand 1980). However, we lack data on the comparative clinical severity of diabetes in New Mexico's ethnic groups, and cannot determine its impact on mortality. Finally, although a large percentage of Hispanics in New Mexico smoke cigarettes, they tend to smoke fewer per day than do non-Hispanic whites (Samet,

Schrag, and Howard 1982; Humble *et al.* 1985). Thus, the effect of smoking on diabetes mortality (Suarez and Barrett-Connor 1984) would be less for Hispanics than for non-Hispanic whites.

A recent survey in New Mexico documents poorer health care for Hispanics with diabetes than for non-Hispanic whites with diabetes (New Mexico Health and Environment Department 1987). Within the last year, 63% of non-Hispanic whites with diabetes had eye examinations, as compared with only 36% of Hispanics with diabetes; and 75% of non-Hispanic whites with diabetes had a foot examination within the past year, as compared with 57% of Hispanics with diabetes. It is not known whether the screening procedures were not offered by the health care providers, or were offered but not performed because of problems with access to care or because of cultural or personal beliefs. Higher diabetes-related hospitalization rates for Hispanics (24%) compared with rates for non-Hispanic whites (4.5%) could reflect an increased severity of disease, and could reflect less timely or less appropriate utilization of health care services by Hispanics.

Health-care beliefs and behavior vary among ethnic groups (Schreiber and Homiak 1981) and may affect diabetes care. Health care usage in San Diego County was found to be lower among persons who spoke only Spanish, when compared with persons who were bilingual (with Spanish as a primary language) or who were primarily English-speaking (Hu and Covell 1986). The difference in health care utilization between these groups was not due to age, income distribution, or lack of bilingual personnel at the health care facilities where the survey was made, but instead may reflect health care beliefs or cultural factors. In the San Antonio Heart Study, Hispanics were noted to be more likely than non-Hispanic whites to express the opinion that Americans are too concerned about losing weight; and Hispanic women scored lower than non-Hispanic women on "sugar avoidance" and "dieting behavior" (Stern *et al.* 1982). These attitudes and behaviors could reduce compliance with recommendations made by health professionals, especially if given by non-Hispanics, and could impede further interaction with a medical care system that continues to emphasize these aspects of care. In addition, when health care messages are delivered in a culturally inappropriate manner, they may be disregarded and the patient may fail to return for further care (Schreiber and Homiak 1981).

Traditional healers (*curanderos* and *curanderas*) continue to play a role in the health care of many Hispanics (Maduro 1983), although their use and influence may be decreasing (Scheper-Hughes and Stewart 1983). Herbs and traditional medicines have been used in the treatment of diabetes (Meyer, Blun, and Cull 1981). However, the effect of these healers or of medicines on diabetes control and complications has not been investigated. All of these considerations may affect health care delivery for Hispanics with diabetes, and thus may ultimately affect mortality.

American Indians
An extremely high prevalence of diabetes has been documented in the Pima Indians (Bennett and Knowler 1979). High prevalence figures are now being documented in other tribes around the country, although they are lower than in the Pima (Gohdes 1986). The prevalence of diabetes in American Indians in New Mexico is also high, with some tribes having a prevalence as high as 31% among adults aged 35 years and older (Carter *et al.* 1989). These high prevalence statistics may be the major factor influencing the high mortality rates we have described among American Indians. It is possible that the rising prevalence observed in the Pima (Bennett and Knowler 1979) is partially responsible for rising mortality rates in American Indians over the 25-year period of our study. Additionally, mortality data for Pima Indians show females with diabetes to have a threefold increase in age-adjusted mortality as compared with nondiabetics; however, no association between diabetes and mortality was noted in males (Pettitt *et al.* 1982).

Although American Indians were once thought to have less complicated diabetes relative to other populations (Prosnitz and Mandell 1967; Saiki and Rimoin 1968), a recent study of the Hopi and Navajo in Arizona found duration-specific complication rates for microvascular disease to be similar to rates in other populations (Rate *et al.* 1983). Additionally, the age-adjusted incidence for American Indians of end-stage renal disease reported to Medicare from 1983 through 1986 was 2.8 times that for whites (Newman *et al.* 1990), and the incidence of lower extremity amputations in diabetic Pima Indians was found to be higher than that reported in other diabetic populations, and to be a risk factor for death (Nelson *et al.* 1988). Cardiovascular disease, however, was found less frequently among Pima Indians than in the general population of Tecumseh, Michigan (Bennett *et al.* 1976). In New Mexico, we have also shown ischemic heart disease mortality to be lower among American Indians than among Hispanics and non-Hispanic whites (Becker *et al.* 1988). This may be due, in part, to the lower smoking rates and to the small number of individuals who smoke heavily among American Indians in New Mexico as compared with other groups (Samet *et al.* 1980; Sievers 1968; DeStefano, Coulehan, and Wiant 1979). The lower prevalence of smoking would be expected to decrease the diabetes mortality among American Indians; however, the higher mortality rates point to other factors as more important determinants.

All American Indians are eligible for primary care through the Indian Health Service (IHS), which has a network of hospitals and clinics throughout New Mexico. However, not all patients are eligible for specialty services when these are not available through the IHS, and the low median income ($9,893) and education level (45.5% completing high school) of American Indians in the state may impede access to these services (U.S. Bureau of the Census 1981). In addition, the constraints imposed by New Mexico's geography are a particular problem for some tribes (Williams 1986). Long distance and poor roads were shown to be health risks for Navajo children in New Mexico who presented to a physician with life-threatening illness (Williams 1987).

Barriers to care may also relate to factors specific to the American Indian cultures of New Mexico. Strong cultural beliefs regarding health and disease are held by many members of American Indian tribes, and traditional healers (Schreiber and Homiak 1981) and herbal remedies have been used for the treatment of diabetes (Meyer, Blun, and Cull 1981); however, no information is available on how these beliefs and activities affect modern diabetes health care. A study conducted among Papago Indians in Arizona found that medicine men and their diagnostic and curing rituals were not in competition with modern medical practice, but addressed different aspects of illness as perceived by the Papago (Shaw 1968). Language barriers to communication with non-Indian providers might affect the quality of health care among the many American Indian tribes in New Mexico, but this potential barrier has not been documented. The perception of a higher body weight as "ideal" among American Plains Indians as compared to the "ideal" among upper-class U.S. white women was noted by West (1974), and could adversely affect diabetes morbidity and mortality. Although generalizations are inappropriate in diverse cultural groups that have significant intertribal variation in health beliefs and practices, such as found in New Mexico, it is possible that barriers to care which are unique to American Indians do affect diabetes mortality.

Our study has several limitations with regard to all three groups. Since there was close agreement in the ICD codes for diabetes during the study period, there should be minimal bias from ICD coding changes. Methodological problems in assessing mortality from diabetes also include age-related development of multi-morbidity (Herman, Teutsch, and Geis 1985), but it is unclear how this would affect the ethnic differences we noted. Our data are limited by using only the underlying cause of death, and not all of the diagnoses listed on the death certificate. This is a potentially serious limitation, as diabetes is selected as the underlying cause of death on only about one-fourth of the certificates where it appears at all and is listed on only about half of the death certificates for persons who have diabetes at the time of death (Harris and Entmacher 1985). The probable impact of ischemic heart disease coding in this regard has been discussed.

Summary

We have demonstrated that New Mexico's American Indian and Hispanic populations have higher diabetes mortality rates than do non-Hispanic whites. While the high prevalence of diabetes in these ethnic groups is a major contributor to these rates, other factors related to the clinical characteristics of diabetes, health care delivery, and self-care practices of the three ethnic groups need to be investigated to develop appropriate and culturally relevant interventions that will improve the health and survival of each of these populations.

REFERENCES

Becker, T. M., C. L. Wiggins, C. R. Key, and J. M. Samet. 1988. Ischemic heart disease mortality in Hispanics, American Indians, and non-Hispanic whites in New Mexico, 1958–1982. *Circulation* 78:302–309.

Bennett, P. H., N. B. Rushforth, M. Miller, and P. M. LeCompte. 1976. Epidemiologic studies of diabetes in the Pima Indians. *Recent Prog.Horm.Res.* 32:333–376.

Bennett, P. H., and W. C. Knowler. 1979. Increasing prevalence of diabetes in the Pima (American) Indians over a ten-year period. In *Proceeding of the 10th Congress of the IDF,* edited by W. K. Waldhause, 507–511. Amsterdam: Excerpta Medica.

Carter, J., R. Horowitz, R. Wilson, S. Sava, P. Sinnock, and D. Gohdes. 1989. Diabetes among American Indians in New Mexico. *Public Health Rep.* 104:665–669.

Centers for Disease Control. 1988. Trends in *diabetes mellitus* mortality. *Morbidity and Mortality Weekly Reports* 37:769–773.

DeStefano, F., J. L. Coulehan, and M. K. Wiant. 1979. Blood pressure survey on the Navajo Indian Reservation. *Am.J.Epidemiol.* 109:335–345.

Diehl, A. K., and M. P. Stern. 1989. Special health problems of Mexican-Americans: obesity, gallbladder disease, *diabetes mellitus,* and cardiovascular disease. *Adv.Intern.Med.* 34:73–96.

Gohdes, D. M. 1986. Diabetes in American Indians: a growing problem. *Diabetes Care* 9:609–613.

Haffner, S. M., M. Rosenthal, H. P. Hazuda, M. P. Stern, and L. J. Franco. 1984.

Evaluation of three potential screening tests for *diabetes mellitus* in a biethnic population. *Diabetes Care* 7:347–353.

Haffner, S. M., D. Fong, and M. P. Stern. 1988. Diabetic retinopathy in Mexican Americans and non-Hispanic whites. *Diabetes* 37:878–884.

Hamman, R. F., G. A. Franklin, E. G. Mayer, S. A. Marshall, J. A. Marshall, J. Baxter, and L. B. Kahn. Microvascular complications of noninsulin-dependent *diabetes mellitus* in Hispanics and whites: the San Luis Valley diabetes study. In *Workshop on diabetes in Hispanics,* May 23–24, 1988, *Program and Abstracts, 13.*

Hamman, R. F., J. A. Marshall, J. Baxter, L. B. Kahn, E. J. Mayer, M. Orleans, J. R. Murphy, and D. C. Legotte. 1989. Methods and prevalence of non-insulin dependent *diabetes mellitus* in a biethnic Colorado population: the San Luis Valley diabetes study. *Am.J.Epidemiol.* 129:295–311.

Harris, M. I., and M. D. Entmacher. 1985. Mortality from diabetes. In *Diabetes in America, National Diabetes Data Group.* DHHS Publication No. (NIH) 85-1468, 1–48. Bethesda, MD: U.S. Government Printing Office.

Herman, W. H., S. M. Teutsch, and L. S. Geis. 1985. Closing the gap: the problem of *diabetes mellitus* in the United States. *Diabetes Care* 8:391–406.

Hu, D. J., and R. M. Covell. 1986. Health care usage by Hispanic outpatients as a function of primary language. In *Cross-cultural medicine. West.J.Med.* 144:490–493.

Humble, C. G., J. M. Samet, D. R. Pathak, and B. J. Skipper. 1985. Cigarette smoking and lung cancer in "Hispanic" whites and other whites in New Mexico. *Am.J.Public Health* 75:145–148.

Maduro, R. 1983. *Curanderismo* and Latino views of disease and curing. *West.J. Med.* 139:863–874.

Meyer, G. C., K. Blun, and J. G. Cull. 1981. *Folk medicine and herbal healing.* Springfield, IL: Charles C. Thomas Publishing.

National Center for Health Statistics. 1960. *Vital statistics of the United States.* Washington, DC: U.S. Government Printing Office.

———. 1965. *Vital statistics of the United States.* Washington, DC: U.S. Government Printing Office.

———. 1970. *Vital statistics of the United States.* Washington, DC: U.S. Government Printing Office.

———. 1975a. *Comparability of mortality statistics for the seventh and eighth revisions of the International Classification of Diseases, United States.* DHEW Publication No. (HRA) 76-1340, 44. Rockville, MD: National Center for Health Statistics.

———. 1975b. *Vital statistics of the United States.* Washington, DC: U.S. Government Printing Office.

———. February 29, 1980a. *Estimates of selected comparability ratios based on dual coding of 1976 death certificates by the eighth and ninth revisions of the International Classification of Diseases.* DHEW Publication No. (PHS) 80-1120, Vol. 28, No. 11, supplement.

———. 1980b. *Vital statistics of the United States.* Washington, DC: U.S. Government Printing Office.

Nelson, R. G., D. M. Gohdes, J. E. Everhart, J. A. Hartner, F. L. Zwemer, D. J. Pettitt, and W. C. Knowler. 1988. Lower extremity amputations in NIDDM: 12-year follow-up study in Pima Indians. *Diabetes Care* 11:8–16.

Newman, J. M., A. A. Marfin, P. W. Eggers, and S. D. Helgerson. 1990. End-stage renal disease among American Indians. *Am.J.Public Health* 80: 318–319.

New Mexico Health and Environment Department. September 1988. *Health for the future: a proposed health policy for New Mexico.* Executive Summary, Recommendations of the Governor's Health Policy Advisory Committee. Santa Fe, NM.

———, Office of Health Promotion. 1987. *New Mexico behavioral risk factor survey, data 1986, diabetes supplement.* Santa Fe, NM.

Nostrand, R. L. 1980. The Hispano homeland in 1990. *Annals of the Association of American Geographers* 70:382–396.

Perez-Stable, E. J., M. M. McMillen, M. I. Harris, R. Z. Juarez, W. C. Knowler, M. P. Stern, and S. G. Haynes. 1989. Self-reported diabetes in Mexican-Americans: Hispanic health and nutrition examination survey, 1982–1984. *Am.J.Public Health* 79:770–772.

Pettit, D. J., J. R. Lisse, W. C. Knowler, and P. H. Bennett. 1982. Mortality as a function of obesity and *diabetes mellitus. Am.J.Epidemiol.* 155:359–366.

Prosnitz, L. R., and G. C. Mandell, 1967. *Diabetes mellitus* among Navajo and Hopi Indians: the lack of vascular complications. *Am.J.Med.Sci.* 253: 700–705.

Pugh, J. A., M. P. Stern, S. M. Haffner, C. W. Eifler, and M. Zapata. 1988. Excess incidence of treatment of end-stage renal disease in Mexican Americans. *Am. J.Epidemiol.* 127:135–144.

Rate, R. G., W. C. Knowler, H. G. Morse, M. D. Bonnell, J. McVey, C. L. Chervenak, M. G. Smith, and G. Pavanich. 1983. *Diabetes mellitus* in Hopi and Navajo Indians: prevalence of microvascular complications. *Diabetes* 32: 894–899.

Roseman, J. M. 1985. Diabetes in black Americans. In *Diabetes in America, National Diabetes Data Group.* DHHS Publication No. (NIH) 85-1468, V:1–7. Bethesda, MD: U.S. Government Printing Office.

Saiki, J. H., and D. C. Rimoin. 1968. *Diabetes mellitus* among the Navajo. In *Clinical features. Arch. Intern. Med.* 122:1–5.

Samet, J. M., C. R. Key, D. M. Kutvirt, and C. L. Wiggins. 1980. Respiratory disease mortality in New Mexico's American Indians and Hispanics. *Am.J. Public Health* 70:492–497.

Samet, J. M., S. D. Schrag, and C. A. Howard. 1982. Respiratory disease in a New Mexico population sample of Hispanic and non-Hispanic whites. *Am. Rev.Respir.Dis.* 125:152–157.

Samet, J. M., D. B. Coultas, C. A. Howard, B. J. Skipper, and C. L. Hanis. 1988. Diabetes, gallbladder disease, obesity and hypertension among Hispanics in New Mexico.*Am.J.Epidemiol.* 128:1302–1311.

Scheper-Hughes, N., and D. Stewart. 1983. *Curanderismo* in Taos County, New

Mexico—a possible case of anthropological romanticism? In *Cross-cultural medicine. West.J.Med.* 139:875–884.
Schreiber, J. M., and J. P. Homiak. 1981. Mexican Americans. In *Ethnicity and medical care*, edited by A. Harwood, 265–335. Cambridge: Harvard University Press.
Shaw, R. D. September 1968. *Health concepts and attitudes of the Papago Indians*. Health Program Systems Center, Division of Indian Health, U.S. Department of Health, Education, and Welfare. Tucson, AZ.
Sievers, M. L. 1968. Cigarette and alcohol usage by southwestern American Indians. *Am.J.Public Health* 58:71–82.
Stern, M. P., and S. P. Gaskill. 1978. Secular trends in ischemic heart disease and stroke mortality. *Circulation* 58:537–543.
Stern, M. P., J. A. Pugh, S. P. Gaskill, and H. P. Hazuda. 1982. Knowledge, attitudes, and behavior related to obesity and dieting in Mexican Americans and Anglos: The San Antonio Heart Study. *Am.J.Epidemiol.* 115:917–928.
Suarez, L., and E. Barrett-Connor. 1984. Interaction between cigarette smoking and *diabetes mellitus* in the prediction of death attributed to cardiovascular disease. *Am.J.Epidemiol.* 120:670–675.
U.S. Bureau of the Census. 1981. Census of the population: 1980. *General Social and Economic Characteristics: New Mexico*. Final Report PC 80-1-C33. Washington, DC: U.S. Government Printing Office.
West, K. M. 1974. Culture, history and adiposity, or should Santa Claus reduce? *Obesity and Bariatric Medicine* 2:48–52.
Williams, J. L. 1986. *New Mexico in maps*. Albuquerque, NM: University of New Mexico Press.
Williams, R. 1987. Meningitis and unpaved roads. *Soc.Sci.Med.* 24:109–115.
World Health Organization. 1957. *Manual of the International Statistical Classification of Diseases, Injuries, and Causes of Death*. Based on the recommendations of the Seventh Revision Conference, 1955. Geneva, Switzerland: WHO.
———. 1967. *Manual of the International Statistical Classification of Diseases, Injuries, and Causes of Death*. Based on the recommendations of the Eighth Revision Conference, 1965. Geneva, Switzerland: WHO.
———. 1977. *Manual of the International Statistical Classification of Diseases, Injuries, and Causes of Death*. Based on the recommendations of the Ninth Revision Conference, 1975. Geneva, Switzerland: WHO.

CHAPTER 5

Infectious Diseases Mortality

Thomas M. Becker
Charles Wiggins
Charles R. Key
Jonathan M. Samet

The nationwide decline in infectious disease mortality over the past century has been well described (Omran 1977; Rosen 1975). Advances in antimicrobial chemotherapy, improvements in sanitation, immunization programs, isolation and quarantine measures, shifts in economic standards, improved nutrition, and increased availability of medical care have all contributed to declining mortality from infectious diseases in the U.S. (Omran 1977; Rosen 1975). For certain infectious diseases, however, the nationwide decline in mortality has been greater among whites than nonwhites (Omran 1977), and the incidence of and mortality from many infectious causes—such as tuberculosis—currently remain higher among nonwhites than whites in the U.S. (Centers for Disease Control [CDC] 1987a, 1987b, 1987c, 1987d).

Trends in infectious disease mortality among some minority groups in the U.S., especially Hispanics and American Indians, have not been adequately examined. The cultural and genetic backgrounds of these populations in New Mexico are distinct, and the state's three ethnic groups have differing prevalences of risk factors for infectious diseases. For example, many American Indians in New Mexico live traditional lifestyles, often in crowded homes with no running water (Becker et al. 1988a). Despite gradual economic improvement in the state over the past quarter century, many disadvantaged minority persons still live in conditions similar to those in developing countries (Ortiz 1979, 1983), with the attendant risks of acquiring many types of infectious diseases. We examined ethnic differences in infectious disease-related mortality in New Mexico for Hispanics, American Indians, and non-Hispanic whites.

Methodologic Considerations

Conforming to International Classification of Diseases (ICD) categories, we examined data for tuberculosis, other (nontuberculous) infections and parasitic diseases, influenza, pneumonia, kidney infections, and meningitis. Because of ICD coding changes, we did not examine diarrheal disease. Case counts were adjusted to the ICD8 coding scheme. The Appendix at the end of this chapter shows the ICD codes we used for these analyses, and indicates the comparability ratios we employed for adjustments of case counts.

Results

The data in Tables 5.1 and 5.2 show substantial differences in infectious disease mortality among New Mexico's three major ethnic populations during the 25-year study period. Age-adjusted mortality rates for most categories of infectious diseases were generally highest among American Indians, followed by Hispanics, for each time period of the study. The greatest differences were evident in most periods for tuberculosis, pneumonia, meningitis, and other infections and parasites, with American Indian rates far exceeding rates for Hispanics and non-Hispanic whites. Ethnic differences for influenza and kidney infections were less striking.

Dramatic declines in mortality rates were observed for American Indians with respect to tuberculosis and other infections and parasites. However, mortality for tuberculosis, pneumonia, meningitis, and other infections and parasites was still higher for American Indians from 1978 through 1982 than for non-Hispanic whites from 1958 through 1962, 25 years earlier. Figures 5.1 through 5.8 present age, period, and cohort graphs for pneumonia among all ethnic and gender groups, and for tuberculosis among American Indians.

Because of elevated mortality rates for infectious causes among young children in New Mexico, we examined age-specific mortality for pneumonia, meningitis, and other infections and parasites by sex and ethnic group among children aged 0 through 4 years. These data show trends similar to the age-adjusted data for non-Hispanic whites, Hispanics, and American Indians in the state, with the highest mortality rates for the American Indian children (Table 5.3).

Discussion

Our data show that the state's three major ethnic populations followed the national trend of decreasing infectious disease-related mortality. The results also indicate substantial ethnic differences in mortality rates from various infectious causes throughout the 25-year study period. For most categories of infections, during each time period age-adjusted mortality rates for American Indians exceeded mortality rates for Hispanics and

Table 5.1
Infection-related mortality rates* in New Mexican males by cause and ethnic group, 1958 through 1982

	Time period (inclusive years)				
	1958–62	1963–67	1968–72	1973–77	1978–82
Tuberculosis					
Non-Hispanic white	9.4	6.5	3.6	2.0	1.0
Hispanic	13.4	9.6	5.1	3.8	3.0
American Indian	40.5	40.5	27.3	23.5	10.7
U.S. white[a]	7.8	5.3	3.3	1.2	1.2
U.S. black[a]	22.6	16.9	12.1	7.1	6.1
Other infections and parasites					
Non-Hispanic white	5.7	4.7	4.9	4.5	6.0
Hispanic	17.6	13.8	9.6	6.7	5.8
American Indian	39.7	44.6	28.0	20.8	15.4
U.S. white[a]	5.5	4.9	5.6	5.6	7.9
U.S. black[a]	16.4	13.2	13.9	14.3	15.6
Influenza					
Non-Hispanic white	2.9	2.3	3.9	4.4	0.9
Hispanic	4.5	2.5	3.0	4.9	1.1
American Indian	8.1	2.2	0.9	5.9	0.0
U.S. white[a]	4.6	1.2	2.1	2.3	1.1
U.S. black[a]	11.2	1.9	3.3	1.7	0.4
Pneumonia					
Non-Hispanic white	34.8	34.3	41.0	42.3	24.8
Hispanic	50.7	44.5	56.9	52.2	36.3
American Indian	88.5	64.5	81.2	89.4	48.3
U.S. white[a]	38.3	36.6	35.1	30.1	28.0
U.S. black[a]	72.6	63.8	61.6	44.3	40.6
Kidney infection					
Non-Hispanic white	3.5	4.0	3.0	1.9	0.7
Hispanic	4.5	5.2	4.6	1.6	1.0
American Indian	10.6	8.6	4.5	1.0	2.5
U.S. white[a]	4.6	5.3	3.8	1.9	0.9
U.S. black[a]	11.0	12.6	9.1	3.8	1.7
Meningitis					
Non-Hispanic white	1.4	1.6	0.5	1.4	0.6
Hispanic	1.2	1.2	0.8	2.1	1.0
American Indian	7.0	10.8	8.2	1.6	2.5
U.S. white[a]	0.7	0.7	0.8	0.8	0.7
U.S. black[a]	2.3	3.2	2.3	2.2	1.8

* Age-adjusted rates per 100,000.
[a] Rates for U.S. whites and blacks are calculated for the midpoints of each 5-year interval (1960, 1965, 1970, 1975, 1980).

Table 5.2
Infection-related mortality rates* in New Mexican females by cause and ethnic group, 1958 through 1982

	Time period (inclusive years)				
	1958–62	1963–67	1968–72	1973–77	1978–82
Tuberculosis					
Non-Hispanic white	3.7	1.7	0.5	0.7	0.8
Hispanic	9.8	4.1	2.2	2.4	1.5
American Indian	38.0	30.1	15.8	12.8	11.6
U.S. white[a]	2.4	1.5	1.0	0.7	0.4
U.S. black[a]	8.8	6.1	4.4	2.7	2.2
Other infections and parasites					
Non-Hispanic white	5.7	4.7	4.9	4.5	6.0
Hispanic	11.9	7.4	7.6	6.4	6.7
American Indian	37.0	38.3	22.5	20.9	12.2
U.S. white[a]	3.5	3.2	4.3	3.9	5.6
U.S. black[a]	9.3	8.5	10.0	10.7	8.4
Influenza					
Non-Hispanic white	2.8	1.2	1.8	3.6	0.7
Hispanic	2.8	3.1	4.7	4.6	0.6
American Indian	4.9	1.5	2.5	3.1	0.7
U.S. white[a]	3.5	1.0	1.5	1.9	1.1
U.S. black[a]	9.0	2.1	2.4	1.2	0.4
Pneumonia					
Non-Hispanic white	19.2	18.7	25.4	26.0	17.0
Hispanic	38.2	32.5	39.9	33.8	22.4
American Indian	65.8	55.0	61.8	47.2	36.9
U.S. white[a]	21.3	22.4	20.8	16.9	17.3
U.S. black[a]	43.7	44.0	40.2	20.9	19.2
Kidney infection					
Non-Hispanic white	2.6	3.6	3.7	1.6	0.7
Hispanic	2.9	6.0	3.8	1.0	0.4
American Indian	12.6	15.4	7.7	4.0	0.0
U.S. white[a]	3.7	4.6	3.5	1.9	1.1
U.S. black[a]	10.1	10.9	7.9	3.3	1.7
Meningitis					
Non-Hispanic white	0.5	1.1	1.0	0.8	0.3
Hispanic	1.1	1.0	1.3	0.7	0.8
American Indian	7.6	8.7	4.4	5.4	3.5
U.S. white[a]	1.0	1.0	0.6	0.6	0.5
U.S. black[a]	3.1	2.4	1.8	1.5	1.3

* Age-adjusted rates per 100,000.
[a] Rates for U.S. whites and blacks are calculated for the midpoints of each 5-year interval (1960, 1965, 1970, 1975, 1980).

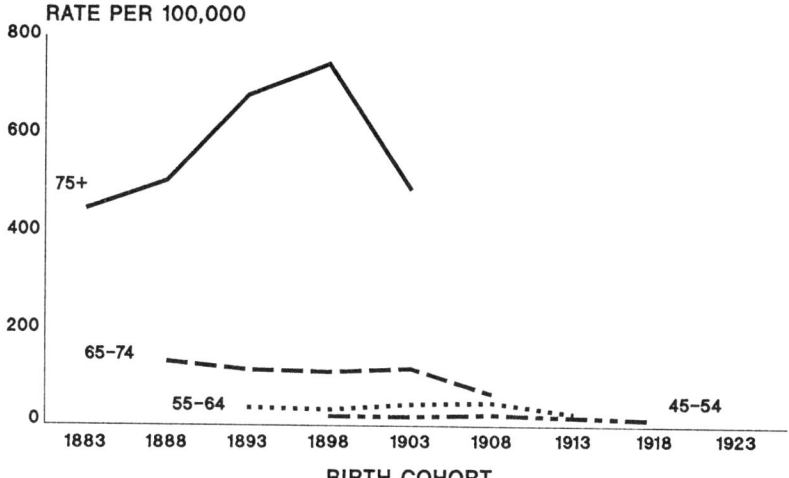

Figure 5.1. *Pneumonia mortality among non-Hispanic white males in New Mexico, by 5-year birth cohort.*

for non-Hispanic whites. The data also show that, for certain infectious causes among American Indians (tuberculosis and meningitis), mortality rates from the most recent period were higher than mortality rates among non-Hispanic whites during the late 1950's and early 1960's.

Few published data describe the incidence of or mortality from infectious diseases among Hispanics in the Southwest. However, an unusually high incidence or prevalence of infectious diseases among southwestern American Indians has been shown for *echinococcus granulosis* (Schantz 1977), plague (Barnes *et al.* 1988), *hemophilus influenzae* infections (Coulehan *et al.* 1984), trachoma (Ludlam 1978), pneumococcal pneumonia (Oseasohn, Skipper, and Tempest 1978), *otitis media* (Johnson 1967; Zonis 1968), genital *chlamydia trachomatis* (Harrison *et al.* 1986), enteric infections (Engleberg *et al.* 1984; Reller 1970), and herpesvirus infections (Becker *et al.* 1988a). Indian Health Service vital statistics also show the high mortality rates for infectious causes among American Indians in the southwest and nationwide (Office of Technology Assessment 1986). Our data support earlier published information on

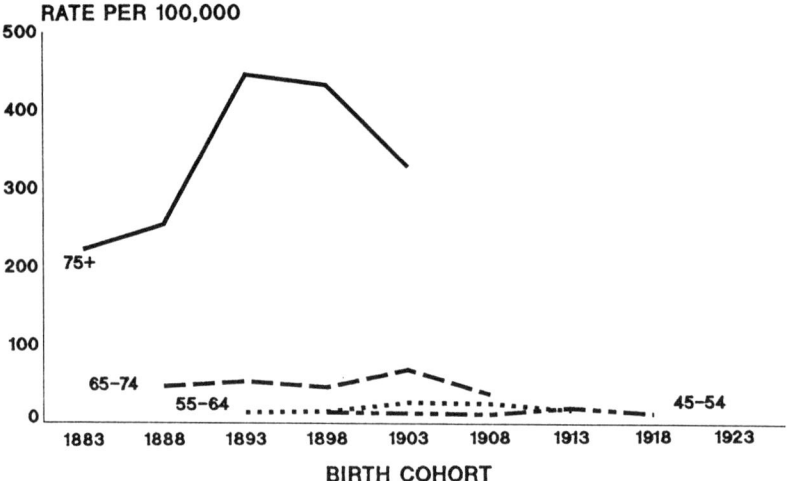

Figure 5.2. *Pneumonia mortality among non-Hispanic white females in New Mexico, by 5-year birth cohort.*

the high infectious-disease-related mortality rates among American Indians, and in addition, provide baseline information on infectious-disease-related mortality among southwestern Hispanics.

Tuberculosis

We observed striking differences in age-adjusted and age-specific mortality rates from tuberculosis among non-Hispanic whites, Hispanics, and American Indians. Several sources have documented high incidence and mortality rates from tuberculosis in American Indians (CDC 1987b; Tempest and Pesanti 1974). In some states, the risk of tuberculosis in 1985 still remained 30-fold higher among American Indians than among other races (CDC 1987b). The prevalence of diabetes, a risk factor for tuberculosis and other infections, is high among southwest American Indians (Bennett, Harris, and Murphy 1982; Bennett *et al.* 1982). Other risks for acquiring tuberculosis among New Mexico's American Indians include crowding in homes (U.S. Bureau of the Census 1982) and high rates of alcoholism (May 1982). For Hispanics nationwide, incidence

INFECTIOUS DISEASES MORTALITY

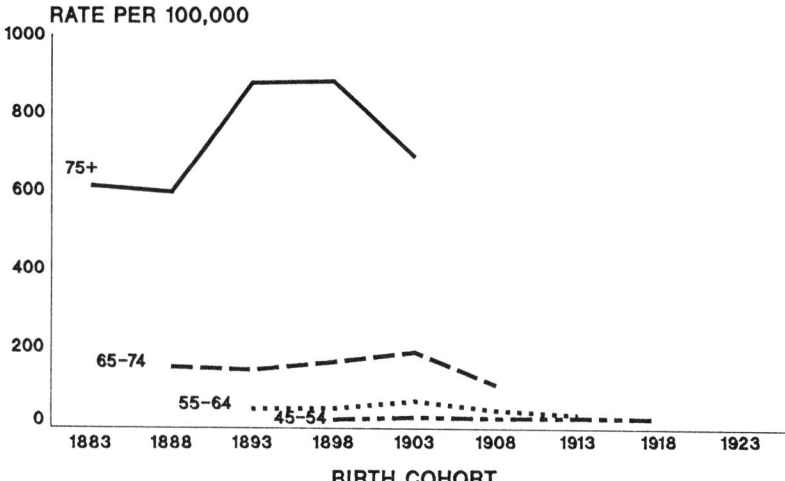

Figure 5.3. *Pneumonia mortality among Hispanic males in New Mexico, by 5-year birth cohort.*

rates for tuberculosis in 1985 were fourfold higher than the national rates for non-Hispanic whites (18.1 per 100,000 *versus* 4.5 per 100,000) (CDC 1987a). Published data on tuberculosis-related mortality for southwestern Hispanics are scant; however, statewide summaries for 1981 through 1983 indicated that Hispanics in New Mexico had a higher mortality rate from tuberculosis than did non-Hispanic whites (New Mexico Health and Environment Department 1985).

Meningitis

Both age-adjusted rates and age-specific rates for children aged 0 through 4 years indicate extraordinarily high mortality from meningitis among American Indians as compared with Hispanics and non-Hispanic whites in New Mexico (Table 5.3). An earlier report based on national data (Feldman, Koehler, and Fraser 1976) has also shown high death rates for meningitis in American Indians, as compared with rates for U.S. whites and blacks, for several etiologic agents, including *N. meningitis, H. influenzae, S. pneumoniae,* and other unspecified agents. For the Navajo in

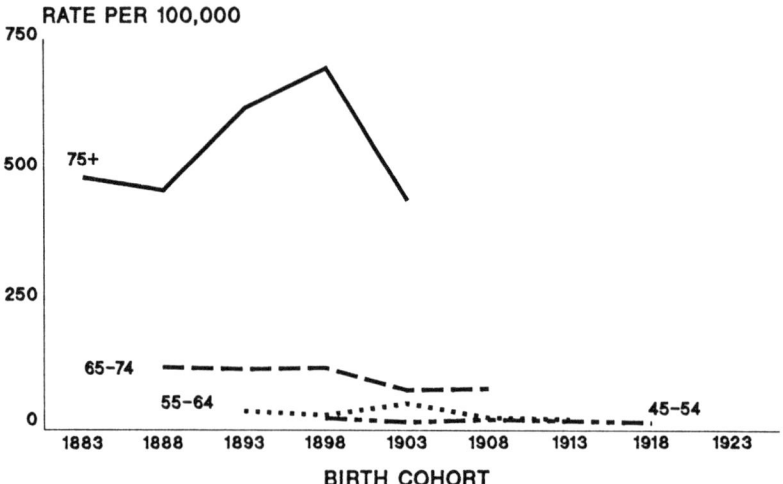

Figure 5.4. *Pneumonia mortality among Hispanic females in New Mexico, by 5-year birth cohort.*

New Mexico and Arizona, the annual incidence rates of *H. influenzae* and pneumococcal meningitis from 1968 through 1980 were much higher than the rates reported from other populations nationwide; however, the case-fatality ratio for *H. influenzae* meningitis in the Navajo was comparable to the national ratio (Coulehan *et al.* 1976, 1984). Other American Indian and Eskimo populations have also demonstrated unusually high rates of *H. influenzae* meningitis. In Arizona, the White Mountain Apache had an eightfold higher incidence of *H. influenzae* meningitis from 1973 through 1981 than was observed nationwide (Losonsky *et al.* 1984), while the Yupik Eskimos and Alaskan Indians had the highest rates of bacterial meningitis yet reported in the United States (84.4 cases per 100,000 population) from 1971 through 1977 (Ward *et al.* 1981). Indian Health Service statistics indicate that the age-adjusted mortality rate from meningitis for the Navajo area from 1980 through 1982 was 4.3-fold higher than the national rate, while for all Indian Health Service areas combined, the rate was 3.6-fold higher than the national rate for all races (Office of Technology Assessment 1986). The high mortality

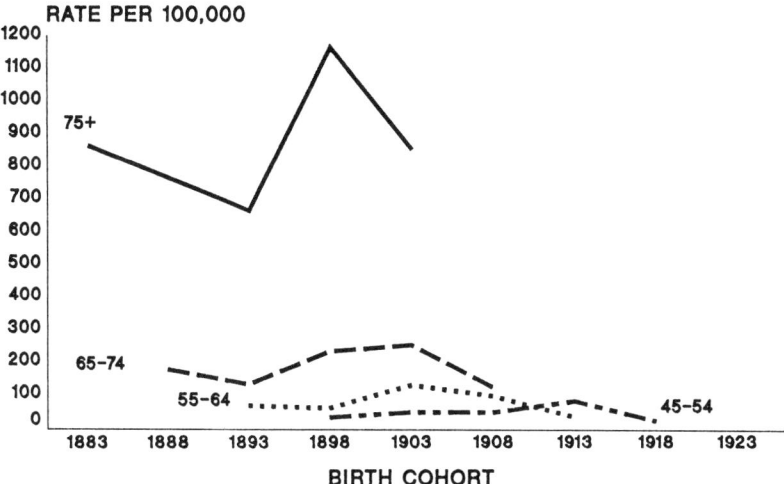

Figure 5.5. *Pneumonia mortality among American Indian males in New Mexico, by 5-year birth cohort.*

rates in American Indians for certain infections—especially pneumococcal, meningococcal, and *H. influenzae* meningitis—may be related to genetic differences in immunologic response to encapsulated organisms (Siber *et al.* 1987; Ward *et al.* 1988; Davidson *et al.* 1989). Although few published data describe incidence or mortality rates for meningitis for southwestern Hispanics, published data for whites (that is Hispanic and non-Hispanic whites combined) in Bernalillo County, New Mexico, indicate that incidence rates for meningitis were comparable to rates for whites in other U.S. cities in the mid-to-late 1960's (Fraser, Geil, and Feldman 1974).

Pneumonia and Influenza

For all races in New Mexico, as for the nation, pneumonia and influenza together are currently the sixth leading cause of death (New Mexico Health and Environment Department 1987). In recent years, pneumonia and influenza combined were the sixth leading cause of death in American Indians in New Mexico, and the eighth leading cause in Hispanics

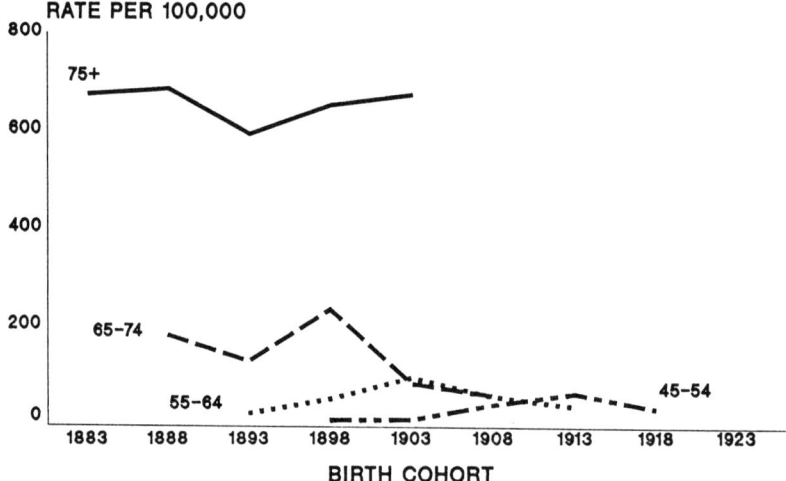

Figure 5.6. *Pneumonia mortality among American Indian females in New Mexico, by 5-year birth cohort.*

(New Mexico Health and Environment Department 1987). Among both Hispanics and non-Hispanic whites from 1983 through 1985, pneumonia and influenza combined accounted for 2.8% of the total proportional mortality (all causes), while 3.4% of American Indian deaths were a result of pneumonia and influenza (New Mexico Health and Environment Department 1987). Indian Health Service statistics for the Navajo area show age-adjusted mortality rates of both pneumonia and influenza that were over two-fold higher than the national rates for all races from 1980 through 1982 (Office of Technology Assessment 1986). Our data show that the age-adjusted mortality rate from pneumonia was higher among both Hispanics and American Indians than among non-Hispanic whites in New Mexico, and higher than the U.S. white rate (Tables 5.2 and 5.3). Oseasohn and coworkers (1978) reported that among the Navajo in New Mexico, incidence rates of pneumonia were high during 1971 and 1972 (1,000 cases per 100,000 persons per year), with a case-fatality ratio of 2.2%. Our age-specific mortality data for pneumonia for children aged 0 through 4 years (Table 5.3) and for adults (Figures 5.1 through 5.6)

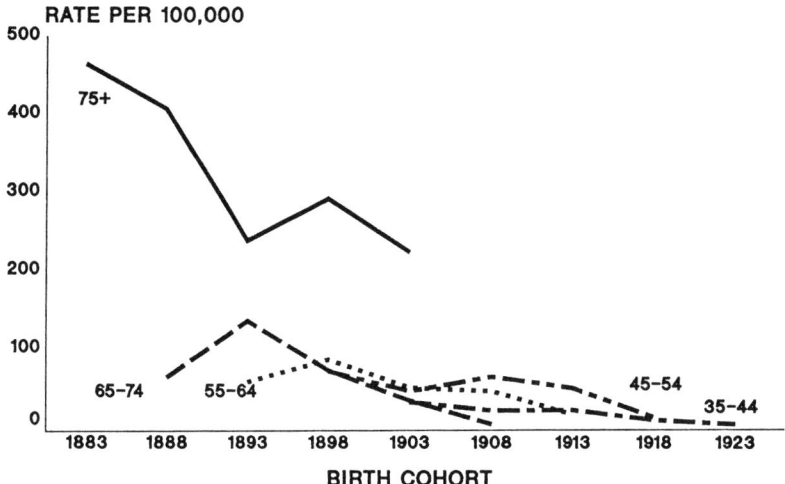

Figure 5.7. *Tuberculosis mortality among American Indian males in New Mexico, by 5-year birth cohort.*

also show higher rates among American Indians and Hispanics than among non-Hispanic whites. As previously suggested, genetic inability to respond immunologically to encapsulated organisms, especially among American Indians, may be closely related to increased mortality from rapidly invasive disease. The age-adjusted rate differences for influenza among the three ethnic populations in this state were less dramatic than the rates for pneumonia, and the small numbers of cases recorded for American Indians may have accounted for the substantial rate variations by time period.

The ethnic differences in infectious-disease-related mortality among Hispanic, American Indian, and non-Hispanic whites in New Mexico may be influenced by the disparate cultural beliefs and medical practices in various communities in the state. Among the Navajo, Pueblo, Zuñi, and Apache tribes, traditional methods of healing by medicine men are still frequently utilized for treatment of a variety of diseases, including infectious diseases (Ortiz 1979, 1983). For American Indians who live a more traditional lifestyle, western medical consultation or treatment may

TUBERCULOSIS MORTALITY
AMERICAN INDIAN FEMALES

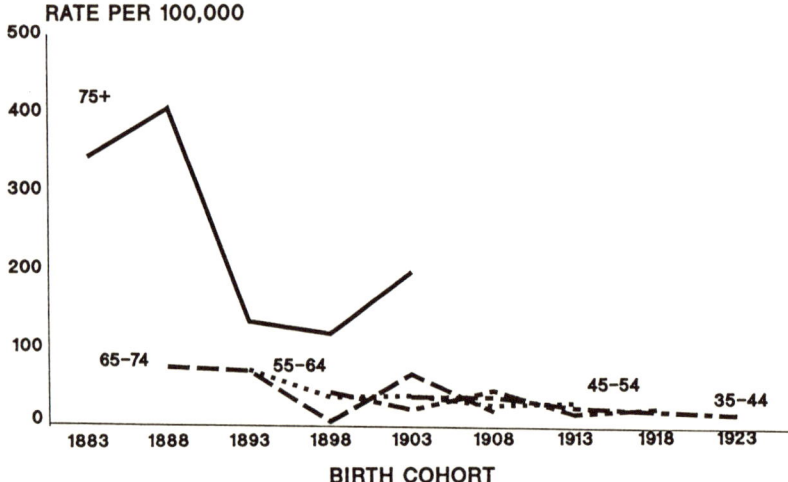

Figure 5.8. *Tuberculosis mortality among American Indian females in New Mexico, by 5-year birth cohort.*

be sought only after the medicine man has been involved in a case. For rapidly invasive infections, such delay in presenting to a hospital can influence mortality. Among Hispanics, the traditional folk healers, *curanderos* and *curanderas,* are commonly consulted for many types of disease (Maduro 1983; Scheper-Hughes and Stewart 1983); and again, delay in seeking Western medical attention could also increase infectious-disease-related mortality rates among Hispanics in New Mexico.

Differences in health care availability in New Mexico may strongly affect mortality rates in the state's various ethnic populations. New Mexico has a large proportion of medically uninsured persons; among Hispanics, the proportion of medically uninsured is higher than among non-Hispanic whites (25% *versus* 13%) (Bennett and Mantlo 1988). Thus, economic constraints affecting availability of health care can influence morbidity and mortality, especially for Hispanics. In addition, many of the rural counties in northern New Mexico are medically underserved (Bennett and Mantlo 1988), especially counties that contain predominant numbers of persons of Hispanic heritage. Lack of health care pro-

Table 5.3
Infection-related mortality rates* in New Mexican children aged 0 through 4 years by cause and ethnic group, 1958 through 1982

	Time period (inclusive years)				
	1958–62	1963–67	1968–72	1973–77	1978–82
Pneumonia					
Males					
Non-Hispanic white	46.0	36.8	30.7	22.8	6.7
Hispanic	131.3	71.0	52.8	23.9	10.5
American Indian	299.8	226.1	150.7	50.0	15.4
Females					
Non-Hispanic white	48.1	35.2	25.6	21.0	6.6
Hispanic	104.2	66.4	46.1	20.4	4.3
American Indian	297.9	151.4	96.4	32.9	10.8
Meningitis					
Males					
Non-Hispanic white	10.7	16.2	3.0	7.3	4.3
Hispanic	5.8	6.4	3.6	10.0	6.5
American Indian	67.3	77.7	59.9	6.7	12.9
Females					
Non-Hispanic white	3.2	7.4	3.2	5.7	2.8
Hispanic	5.1	8.5	9.4	1.7	4.1
American Indian	50.5	65.8	29.6	29.6	9.2
Other infections and parasites					
Males					
Non-Hispanic white	22.1	18.5	13.2	11.0	4.6
Hispanic	110.8	60.7	26.8	16.5	16.0
American Indian	323.8	290.6	166.8	80.0	30.5
Females					
Non-Hispanic white	23.1	11.2	12.7	11.5	11.0
Hispanic	98.5	39.9	30.7	18.7	11.6
American Indian	246.9	197.0	98.0	72.4	16.1

* Age-specific rates per 100,000.

viders in these areas also affects infectious disease morbidity and mortality. Although the Indian Health Service provides care at no cost to New Mexico's American Indians, geographic barriers—including long distances to hospitals and travel over unimproved roads (Williams 1987)—can strongly influence health care availability for American Indians. Williams has recently demonstrated that among the Navajo, travel on unpaved roads was a risk factor for children presenting with bacterial meningitis as compared to those presenting with less severe forms of infections (Williams 1987).

In addition to differences in availability and utilization of health care, minorities in New Mexico may have higher mortality rates from infections than do non-Hispanic whites for other reasons. It is not known whether the incidence of infections is higher in minorities than in the majority (non-Hispanic white) population, with case fatality ratios that are similar in both groups; or whether the incidence of infections is comparable in both groups, but the case-fatality ratios are higher in minorities. It is possible, also, that both incidence and case-fatality ratios are higher in minorities than in non-Hispanic whites. Unfortunately, few published studies have directly addressed these issues among the various minority groups nationwide, and a population-based perspective on infectious disease incidence and mortality has been underemphasized.

Our analyses of vital data have several limitations that have been discussed in detail in other publications (Becker *et al.* 1988b; Samet *et al.* 1988) and in earlier chapters of this text. We need to caution, moreover, that bias may enter this study from the changes in the ICD codes for various infectious diseases. Our adjustments in the classification of infectious disease mortality were designed to reduce artifactual changes in mortality rates caused by inconsistencies in the coding schemes spanning the seventh, eighth, and ninth ICD revisions. Although the adjustments among various ICD revisions may bias our results toward the null (that is, no recent decline in infectious disease mortality in New Mexico), our data still revealed a declining trend in infectious disease mortality for all ethnic groups during the 25-year period of this study. From the public health perspective, however, our data emphasize the importance of targeting the state's high-risk minority populations with a view towards providing timely and appropriate medical care—including vaccination—to reduce mortality from infectious causes in New Mexico.

Summary

We observed declining mortality from most infectious causes in each ethnic and gender group in New Mexico throughout the 25-year study period. The greatest ethnic differences in mortality rates were evident for tuberculosis, pneumonia, meningitis, and for other infections and parasites, with American Indians demonstrating elevated rates as compared with the non-Indian populations of the state. Age-specific data for American Indian children 0 through 4 years showed dramatic decreases in mortality rates from the earliest to the most recent periods for pneumonia, meningitis, and for other infections and parasites. Nonetheless, despite the improvements in mortality from infectious diseases in each ethnic group in this state, minority populations in New Mexico remain at increased risk of dying from infectious causes.

Appendix

Comparability ratios for infectious diseases in the seventh, eighth, and ninth revisions of the International Classification of Diseases *

Cause of death	8th Revision ICD Code No.	Comparability ratio between ICD8 and ICD7 [a]	Comparability ratio between ICD8 and ICD9 [b]
Tuberculosis	010–019	0.950	1.304
Other infectious and parasitic diseases	Remainder of 000–136	0.924	1.196
Meningitis	320	0.959	1.057
Influenza	470–474	0.960	1.030
Pneumonia	480–486	0.994	1.096
Kidney infection	590	1.026	1.002

* World Health Organization 1957, 1967, 1977.
[a] Ratio expressed as ICD8:ICD7.
[b] Ratio expressed as ICD8:ICD9.

REFERENCES

Barnes, A. M., T. J. Quan, M. L. Beard, and G. O. Maupin. 1988. Plague in American Indians, 1956–1987. *Morbidity and Mortality Weekly Reports* 37:11–16.

Becker, T. M., L. S. Madger, H. R. Harrison, J. Stewart, D. D. Humphrey, J. Hauler, and A. J. Nahmias. 1988a. The epidemiology of infection with the human herpesvirus in Navajo children. *Am.J.Epidemiol.* 127:1071–1078.

Becker, T. M., C. L. Wiggins, C. R. Key, and J. M. Samet. 1988b. Ischemic heart disease mortality in Hispanics, American Indians, and non-Hispanic whites in New Mexico, 1958–1982. *Circulation* 78:302–309.

Bennett, P. H., M. Harris, and R. S. Murphy. 1982. Geographic and ethnic differences in diabetes frequency in the Americas. In *Diabetes 1982: Proceedings of the 11th Congress of the International Diabetes Federation*, edited by E. N. Mongola. Amsterdam-Oxford-Princeton: *Excerpta Medica*.

Bennett, P. H., W. C. Knowler, D. J. Pettit, M. J. Carraher, and B. Vasquez. 1982. Longitudinal studies of the development of diabetes in the Pima Indians. In *Advances in diabetes epidemiology*, edited by E. Eschewege. Amsterdam: Elsevier Press.

Bennett, M., and E. J. Mantlo. 1988. *New Mexico Resources Registry, Statistical Summary 1986–87*. Albuquerque, NM: University of New Mexico Medical Center Press.

Centers for Disease Control. 1987a. Tuberculosis among Hispanics—United States. *Morbidity and Mortality Weekly Reports* 36:568–569.

———. 1987b. Tuberculosis among American Indians and Alaska Natives—United States. *Morbidity and Mortality Weekly Reports* 36:493–495.

———. 1987c. Tuberculosis in minorities—United States. *Morbidity and Mortality Weekly Reports* 36:77–80.

———. 1987d. Tuberculosis among Asians/Pacific Islanders—United States. *Morbidity and Mortality Weekly Reports* 36:331–334.

Coulehan, J. L., R. H. Michaels, K. E. Williams, D. K. Lemley, C. P. North, T. K. Welty, and K. D. Rogers. 1976. Bacterial meningitis in Navajo Indians. *Public Health Rep.* 91:4644–4648.

Coulehan, J. L., R. D. Michaels, C. Hallowell, R. Schults, T. K. Welty, and J. S. C. Kno. 1984. Epidemiology of *Haemophilus influenza* Type B disease among Navajo Indians. *Public Health Rep.* 99:404–409.

Davidson, M., C. D. Schraer, A. J. Parkinson, J. F. Campbell, R. R. Facklam, R. B. Wainwright, A. P. Lanier, and W. L. Heyward. January 1989. *Invasive pneumoccal disease in an Alaska Native population*. Abstract. Indian Health Service Research Conference, Tucson, AZ.

Engleberg, N. C., A. Correa-Villasenor, C. Q. North, T. Crow, J. G. Wells, and P. A. Blake. Campylobacter enteritis on Hopi and Navajo Indian Reservations. 1984. *West.J.Med.* 141:53–56.

Feldman, R. A., R. E. Koehler, and D. W. Fraser. 1976. Race-specific differences in bacterial meningitis death in the United States, 1962–1968. *Am.J.Public Health* 66:392–396.

Fraser, D. W., C. C. Geil, and R. A. Feldman. 1974. Bacterial meningitis in Bernalillo County, New Mexico: a comparison with three other American populations. *Am.J.Epidemiol.* 100:29–34.

Harrison, H. R., L. S. Madger, W. T. Boyce, J. Hauler, T. M. Becker, J. A. Stewart, and D. D. Humphrey. 1986. Acute *chlamydia trachomatis* respiratory infection in childhood: serologic evidence. *Am.J.Dis. Child.* 140:1068–1071.

Johnson, R. L. 1967. Chronic *otitis media* in school age Navajo Indians. *Laryngoscope* 7:1900–1995.

Losonsky, G. A., M. Santosham, V. M. Sehgal, A. Zwalen, and E. R. Moxon.

1984. *Haemophilus influenza* disease in the White Mountain Apaches: molecular epidemiology of high risk population. *Pediatr.Infec.Dis.* 3:539–547.

Ludlam, J. A. 1978. Prevalence of trachoma among Navajo Indian children. *Am.J.Optom.Physiol.Opt.* 55:116–118.

Maduro, R. 1983. *Curanderismo* and Latino views of disease and curing. *West.J.Med.* 139:863–874.

May, P. A. 1982. Substance abuse and American Indians: prevalence and susceptibility. *Int.J.Addictions* 17:1185–1209.

New Mexico Health and Environment Department. 1985. *Selected health statistics, New Mexico, 1982–83*. Health Services Division, Santa Fe, NM.

———. *Selected health statistics, New Mexico, 1985*. 1987. Health Services Division, Santa Fe, NM.

Office of Technology Assessment. April 1986. *Indian health care*. OTA-H-290. Washington, DC: U.S. Government Printing Office.

Omran, A. R. 1977. Epidemiologic transition in the United States. *Population Bulletin* 32:3–45.

Ortiz, A., ed. 1979. *Handbook of North American Indians*. Vol. 9, *Southwest*. Smithsonian Institution. Washington, DC: U.S. Government Printing Office.

———, ed. 1983. *Handbook of North American Indians*. Vol. 10, *Southwest*. Smithsonian Institution. Washington, DC: U.S. Government Printing Office.

Oseasohn, R., B. E. Skipper, and B. Tempest. 1978. Pneumonia in a Navajo community. *Am.Rev.Respir.Dis.* 117:1003–1009.

Reller, L. B., and M. I. Spector. 1970. Shigellosis among Indians. *J.Infect.Dis.* 121:355–357.

Rosen, G. 1975. *Preventive medicine in the United States 1900–1975*. New York: Science History Publications.

Samet, J. M., C. L. Wiggins, C. R. Key, and T. M. Becker. 1988. Mortality for lung cancer and COPD in New Mexico, 1958–82. *Am.J.Public Health* 78:1182–1186.

Schantz, P. M. 1977. *Echinococcus* in American Indians living in Arizona and New Mexico. *Am.J.Epidemiol.* 106:370–379.

Scheper-Hughes, N., and D. Stewart. 1983. *Curanderismo* in Taos County, New Mexico—possible case of anthropological romanticism. *West.J.Med.* 139:875–884.

Siber, G. R., M. Santosham, C. M. Priehs, R. Reid, W. Letson, D. Madore, and R. Eby. October 1987. *Impaired antibody response to H. influenza b capsular polysaccharide in Native American children*. Abstract 326. New York: ICAAC.

Tempest, B., and E. Pesanti. 1974. A community-wide tuberculosis case finding program on the Navajo Reservation. *Am.Rev.Respir.Dis.* 110:760–764.

U.S. Bureau of the Census. 1982. *Census of population: 1980. General population characteristics. Final report. New Mexico*. PC80-1-B33. Washington, DC: U.S. Government Printing Office.

Ward, J. I., H. S. Margolis, M. K. W. Lum, D. W. Fraser, and T. R. Bender. 1981. *Haemophilus influenza* disease in Alaskan Eskimos: characteristics of a population with an unusual incidence of invasive disease. *Lancet* June: 1281–1285.

Ward, J. I., G. Brenneman, G. Letson, and W. Heyward. 1988. *Limited protective efficacy of an H. influenza type b conjugate vaccine in Native Alaskan infants immunized at 2, 4, and 6 months of age.* Abstract 1127. New Orleans: ICAAC.

Williams, R. 1987. Meningitis and unpaved roads. *Soc.Sci.Med.* 24:109–115.

World Health Organization. 1957. *Manual of the International Statistical Classification of Diseases, Injuries, and Causes of Death.* Based on the recommendations of the Seventh Revision Conference, 1955. Geneva, Switzerland: WHO.

———. 1967. *Manual of the International Statistical Classification of Diseases, Injuries, and Causes of Death.* Based on the recommendations of the Eighth Revision Conference, 1965. Geneva, Switzerland: WHO.

———. 1977. *Manual of the International Statistical Classification of Diseases, Injuries, and Causes of Death.* Based on the recommendations of the Ninth Revision Conference, 1975. Geneva, Switzerland: WHO.

Zonis, R. D. 1968. Chronic *otitis media* in the southwestern American Indian. *Arch.Otolaryngol.* 88:40–45.

CHAPTER 6

Ischemic Heart Disease Mortality

Thomas M. Becker
Charles Wiggins
Charles R. Key
Jonathan M. Samet

The rise and fall of ischemic heart disease mortality in the U.S. over the last 25 years has been well documented (Stallones 1980). It is not clear, however, whether all racial and ethnic groups have shared in the nationwide decrease in mortality from ischemic heart disease of recent years. Mortality from ischemic heart disease in Hispanics and American Indians—the principal minority groups in the Southwest—has not been adequately examined. Although a low prevalence of coronary artery disease in southwestern American Indians has been reported, most of the documentation has been from case reports, postmortem anatomic studies, and population surveys that were limited by short observation periods (Sievers 1966, 1967; Salsbury 1937; Kraus 1954; Gilbert 1955; Smith, Salsbury, and Gilliam 1956). Among southwestern Hispanics, long-term trends in ischemic heart disease mortality have not been well described.

To examine ethnic differences in ischemic heart disease mortality in the three major ethnic groups in New Mexico, and to determine whether trends in mortality in these populations followed recent nationwide decreases, we analyzed vital records data collected from 1958 through 1982.

Methodologic Considerations

We obtained coded death certificate data for residents of New Mexico for the years 1958 through 1982 from the New Mexico Bureau of Vital Statistics. Cause of death was coded according to the seventh revision of the International Classification of Diseases (ICD) for 1958 through 1968 (World Health Organization [WHO] 1957), the eighth ICD revision for 1969 through 1978 (WHO 1967), and the ninth ICD revision for 1979 through 1982 (WHO 1977). For this report, deaths attributed to ischemic heart disease included ICD 420–420.9, 422.1, 440, 441, and 443 in the seventh revision; ICD 410–413 in the eighth revision; and ICD 410–414.9 in the ninth revision.

We adjusted all ischemic heart disease deaths recorded over the 25-year study period to the coding scheme of the eighth ICD revision. Changes in coding procedures for ischemic heart disease in 1969 resulted in the assignment of more deaths to this category than had been assigned to the most nearly comparable category—"arteriosclerotic heart disease, including coronary artery disease"—in the seventh revision (U.S. Department of Health, Education, and Welfare 1979). The resulting comparability ratio of 1.146 expresses the differences in coding changes between ICD revisions seven and eight (Salsbury 1937). A comparability ratio of 0.998 results if ischemic heart disease (ICD 410–413, eighth revision) is compared with the following combined categories in ICD seventh revision: "arteriosclerotic heart disease, including coronary disease" (ICD 420); "other myocardial degeneration with arteriosclerosis" (ICD 422.1) and "other hypertensive heart disease" (ICD 440, 441, 443) (U.S. Department of Health, Education, and Welfare 1979). To control for artifactual elevation of ischemic heart disease mortality rates associated with coding changes, we included this combination of ischemic heart disease mortality codes from the seventh revision in our rate calculations for 1958 through 1968; this grouping more closely approximated the changed coding of cardiovascular mortality in the eighth ICD revision.

We also adjusted the mortality figures for 1979 through 1982, coded under the ninth ICD revision, to make them more comparable with data coded under the eighth revision for ischemic heart disease. We calculated age-specific and age-adjusted mortality rates for 1979 through 1982 by dividing the numbers of cases during these years by 0.8784, the comparability ratio for ischemic heart disease mortality between the ninth and the eighth ICD revisions. This ratio was used by Sorlie and Gold (1987) in a study of the impact of the change from the eighth to the ninth ICD coding scheme. Adjustment by this ratio reduces artifactual decreases in ischemic heart disease mortality that would result from the incomparability of the ICD codes when the ninth ICD revision went into effect in 1979 (Sorlie and Gold 1987).

Results

Striking differences in ischemic heart disease mortality were evident among New Mexico's three major ethnic populations during the 25-year study period (Table 6.1). Age-adjusted mortality rates from ischemic heart disease among Hispanics and among non-Hispanic white men

Table 6.1
Mortality rates* in New Mexicans from ischemic heart disease, 1958 through 1982

	Time period (inclusive years)				
	1958–62	1963–67	1968–72	1973–77	1978–82
Males					
Non-Hispanic white	301.1	302.5	318.9	282.5	231.4
Hispanic	167.2	195.6	224.5	187.1	159.8
American Indian	95.0	74.4	101.7	98.4	76.6
U.S. white	461.2	501.2	443.8	395.4	352.9
Females					
Non-Hispanic white	142.9	123.0	142.2	127.4	109.8
Hispanic	121.8	133.9	139.4	104.9	91.6
American Indian	44.8	63.0	59.2	39.4	28.3
U.S. white	261.5	279.1	234.3	205.7	184.1

* Age-adjusted rates per 100,000.

showed comparable increases from the first to the third time periods, followed by decreasing rates from 1973 through 1982. American Indian men also showed a peak in ischemic heart disease mortality in 1970, followed by a decline in rates, although the pattern of increasing mortality rates was not observed from 1958 through 1968. Among American Indian women, the decline in ischemic heart disease mortality occurred earlier, after the 1963 through 1967 time period. Among non-Hispanic white women, comparable peaks in ischemic heart disease mortality rates were observed from 1958 through 1962 and from 1968 through 1972; declining rates were observed from 1973 through 1982.

The age-adjusted ischemic heart disease mortality rates for Hispanics of both sexes were lower than for non-Hispanic whites, except for Hispanic women from 1963 through 1967. Differences in mortality rates between Hispanics and non-Hispanic whites were more pronounced for men than for women in each 5-year period from 1958 through 1982. Hispanic mortality rates for ischemic heart disease exceeded rates for American Indians in every time period. The age-adjusted ischemic heart disease mortality rates for American Indians were one-fourth to one-half the rates for New Mexico's non-Hispanic whites. The age-adjusted mortality rates from ischemic heart disease in non-Hispanic whites in New Mexico were lower than national rates for whites.

When data were examined by 5-year birth cohorts spanning the years

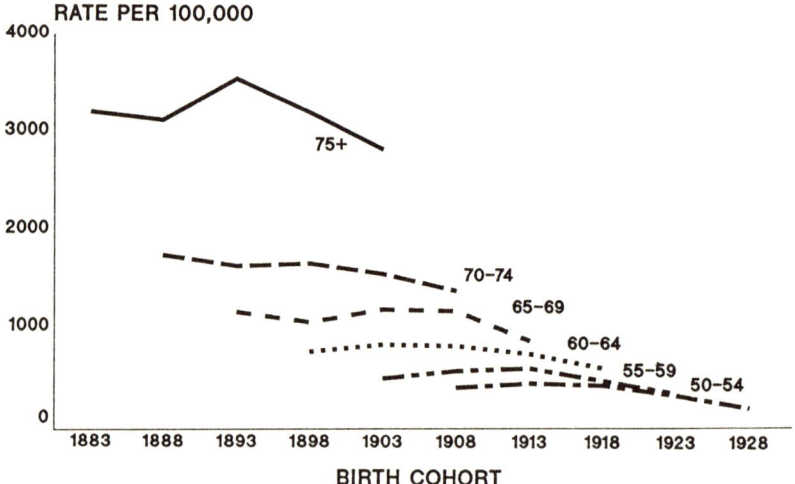

Figure 6.1. *Ischemic heart disease mortality in non-Hispanic white males in New Mexico, by 5-year birth cohort.*

1885 through 1920, the rise-and-fall pattern of age-specific mortality from ischemic heart disease was observed in most age groups in non-Hispanic whites, Hispanics, and American Indians (Figures 6.1 through 6.6). Among the three ethnic groups, the rise-and-fall patterns of age-specific mortality were most clearly observed in the oldest age groups of Hispanics and non-Hispanic whites.

Discussion

Our analysis of vital statistics data for New Mexico shows that the state's three major ethnic groups—non-Hispanic whites, Hispanics, and American Indians—followed the national trend of decreasing ischemic heart disease mortality. The results also indicate low mortality rates from ischemic heart disease for New Mexico's principal minority groups. Furthermore, our study reaffirms that mortality rates for ischemic heart disease

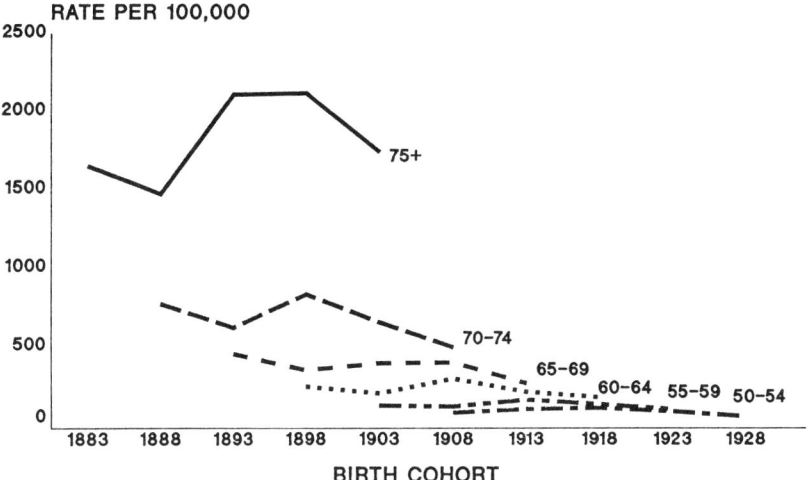

Figure 6.2. *Ischemic heart disease mortality in non-Hispanic white females in New Mexico, by 5-year birth cohort.*

in New Mexico's non-Hispanic whites are lower than the rates for whites nationwide (Stallones 1980).

We found that Hispanics in New Mexico are at lower risk than non-Hispanic whites for death from ischemic heart disease. Our findings are in accord with other research, which also has shown southwestern Hispanics to be at lower risk than non-Hispanics for ischemic heart disease mortality. In Bexar County, Texas, Hispanics (especially men) had lower mortality rates from ischemic heart disease than did non-Hispanics in the years 1970 through 1976 (Stern et al., in press); statewide in Texas, Hispanic men had lower mortality rates from ischemic heart disease than did non-Hispanics in the years 1970 and 1980 (Stern et al. 1987). In California, Hispanic men had lower mortality from all cardiovascular causes than did non-Hispanic men, although rates in Hispanic women were comparable with those of non-Hispanic women during the 1969 through 1971 study period (Schoen and Nelson 1981). In Orange County, California, Hispanics had lower mortality rates in 1978 from all diseases of

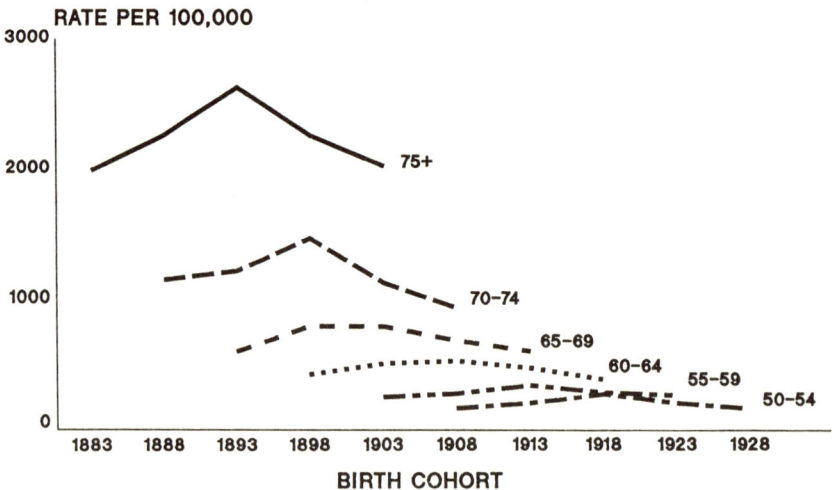

Figure 6.3. *Ischemic heart disease mortality in Hispanic males in New Mexico, by 5-year birth cohort.*

the heart than did non-Hispanic whites (Schoen and Nelson 1981). In an earlier report from New Mexico for 1972 through 1974, ischemic heart disease mortality for Hispanic men ranged from 25% to 40% lower than for non-Hispanic men (Buechley *et al.* 1979).

Comparable with observations in Texas (Stern and Gaskill 1978; Stern *et al.* 1987), our study showed that differences in age-adjusted mortality rates between Hispanic and non-Hispanic whites were greater for men than for women over the entire 25-year study period (Table 6.1). For men, these differences were greater in New Mexico than in Texas (Stern *et al.* 1987): in 1970 and 1980, mortality rates for Hispanic men were approximately 30% lower in New Mexico and approximately 15% lower in Texas. Comparable with observations in Texas, our data for New Mexico showed declining ischemic heart disease mortality in Hispanics in recent years (Stern *et al.* 1987, in press). In Hispanic men in New Mexico, however, the decline in ischemic heart disease mortality from the peak period (1968 through 1972) to the most recent period (1978 through 1982) paralleled the decline observed in non-Hispanic white men (27%

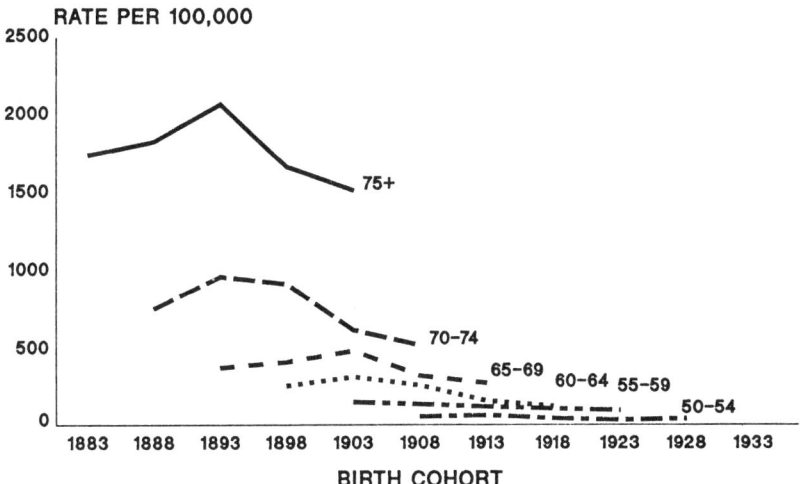

Figure 6.4. *Ischemic heart disease mortality in Hispanic females in New Mexico, by 5-year birth cohort.*

to 29%) (Table 6.1). In Hispanic men in Texas, ischemic heart disease mortality declined at approximately one-half the rate it declined in non-Hispanic men over the same period (Stern *et al.* 1987). In Hispanic women in New Mexico, the rate of decline was steeper from the peak period to the most recent period (34%) than in non-Hispanic white women during the same years (23%) (Table 6.1). These data contrast with the data in Texas, which indicated comparable declines for Hispanic and non-Hispanic white women from 1970 through 1980 (Stern *et al.* 1987).

Available data on risk factors do not adequately explain the lower rates of ischemic heart disease mortality among Hispanics. Both serum cholesterol levels and serum triglycerides appear to be comparable between Hispanics and non-Hispanic whites (Kraus, Borhani, and Franti 1980; Friis *et al.* 1981; Stern *et al.* 1984). The San Antonio Heart Study showed few ethnic differences between Hispanics and non-Hispanics with regard to lipoprotein profiles, although Hispanic women of lower socioeconomic status had a lower level of high-density lipoproteins (Stern *et al.* 1984). Population surveys in Texas and New Mexico showed that a higher pro-

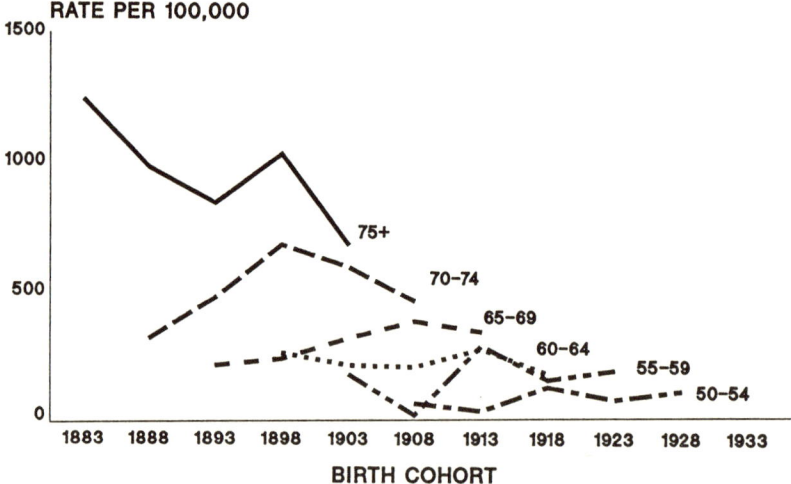

Figure 6.5. *Ischemic heart disease mortality in American Indian males in New Mexico, by 5-year birth cohort.*

portion of Hispanics than non-Hispanics were obese (Stern *et al.* 1982a, 1984, 1985; Mueller *et al.* 1984; New Mexico Health and Environment Department 1987; Samet *et al.* 1988). Hispanics in Texas also showed a higher prevalence of type 2 diabetes than did non-Hispanics (Hanis *et al.* 1983; Gardner *et al.* 1984; Stern *et al.* 1985), and Hispanic men showed a higher prevalence of hypertension, although Hispanic women showed a lower prevalence of hypertension (Stern *et al.* 1982b). More recent research in Texas, however, revealed that the prevalence of hypertension among Hispanic men was similar to that among non-Hispanic white men; the prevalence among Hispanic women remained lower than among non-Hispanic white women (Franco *et al.* 1985). The Behavioral Risk Factor Survey in New Mexico demonstrated comparable proportions of hypertensive Hispanics and non-Hispanic whites (New Mexico Health and Environment Department 1987). A recent survey of an Hispanic community near Albuquerque, New Mexico, also revealed no excess of hypertensive adults (Samet *et al.* 1988). In addition, cigarette smoking in Hispanic men is as common as in non-Hispanic whites (Samet *et al.*

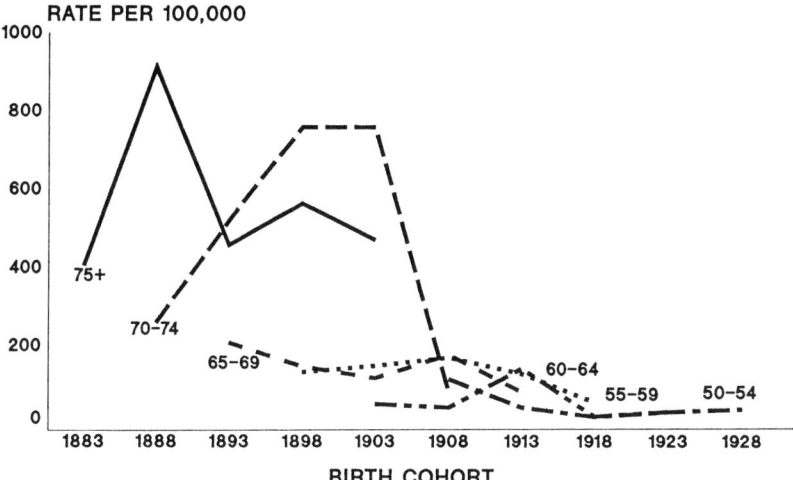

Figure 6.6. *Ischemic heart disease mortality in American Indian females in New Mexico, by 5-year birth cohort.*

1982; Marcus and Crane 1985; New Mexico Health and Environment Department 1987; Markides, Coreil, and Ray 1987), although the numbers of cigarettes smoked per day tends to be less among Hispanics. Dietary factors, patterns of alcohol use, physical activity, and stress have not been adequately evaluated as cardiovascular disease risk factors in New Mexico's Hispanics.

We also observed low rates of ischemic heart disease mortality in American Indians in New Mexico. Other reports have previously documented low rates of ischemic heart disease-related mortality in southwestern American Indians. Mortality data compiled by the Indian Health Service (Office of Technology and Assessment 1986) indicate that within certain health service areas in New Mexico, heart disease mortality in American Indians remains the second leading cause of death, although rates are comparatively low and decreased from 1972 through 1982. The Albuquerque Area Indian Health Service facilities serve approximately 40% of New Mexico's American Indians; in this service area, the mortality rates from ischemic heart disease from 1980 through 1982 were less than one-third the national rate. In the Navajo Area, mortality rates for the same period were one-fifth the national rate. The low mortality from ischemic heart disease among American Indians in New Mexico is not characteristic of all American Indian tribes, however, as several northwestern, midwestern, and eastern tribes have ischemic heart disease mortality rates that exceed national rates (Office of Technology and Assessment 1986).

Risk factors for ischemic heart disease in most of the American Indian tribes have not been described, although some observations on risk factors provide several potential explanations for the low rates of mortality from ischemic heart disease among American Indians in New Mexico. Members of southwestern tribes have lower plasma cholesterol levels than do age- and weight-matched whites; furthermore, the levels rise very little with advancing age (Sievers 1968a; Sievers and Fisher 1979). Southwestern Indians also have a higher ratio of high-density lipoproteins to low-density lipoproteins as compared with non-Indian controls (Garnick, Bennett, and Langer 1979). In addition, southwestern Indians rarely smoke cigarettes, and very few individuals smoke heavily (Sievers 1968b; DeStafano, Coulehan, and Wiant 1979; Samet *et al.* 1980). However, the prevalence of diabetes and obesity in southwestern American Indians is much higher than in U.S. whites (West 1974, 1978; Sievers 1976; Knowler *et al.* 1981; U.S. Department of Health and Human Services 1983), and rates of hypertension are also higher than in U.S. whites (Sievers 1966, 1977). Among the Navajo, the major risk factors for acute myocardial infarction include hypertension, diabetes, and obesity (Coulehan *et al.* 1986). Although it has been suggested that low levels of interpersonal competitiveness and stress in southwestern Indians are a factor in low rates of ischemic heart disease (Sievers 1967), the data are not convincing. Stress as a cardiovascular risk factor in Indians needs to be addressed more thoroughly. Dietary factors, patterns of alcohol use, and physical activity also warrant evaluation as cardiac disease risk factors in southwestern Indians.

In addition to published information on ischemic heart disease mortality in American Indians, available data on morbidity from ischemia also indicate low rates in southwestern tribes. Acute myocardial infarction in southwestern American Indians occurs at rates much lower than nationwide (Coulehan 1986; Sievers and Fisher 1979). Sievers and Fisher (1979) observed an increasing frequency of acute myocardial infarction in southwestern Indian tribes from 1957 through 1978, but acute myocardial infarction occurred at only one-fifth the national rate. Among the Navajo, rates for acute myocardial infarction were one-fourth to one-fifth the national rate (Coulehan *et al.* 1986). Targeted investigations of acute myocardial infarction among the Pueblo and Apache tribes, who constitute a large proportion of New Mexico's Indian population, have not been reported.

We observed lower rates of mortality from ischemic heart disease among New Mexico's non-Hispanic whites than among U.S. whites. Previous studies have also shown lower mortality rates from ischemic heart disease in non-Hispanic whites in New Mexico than in whites nationwide (Buechley et al. 1979; Stallones 1980). Other western states with populations composed mostly of non-Hispanic whites also show lower mortality rates for ischemic heart disease than are observed nationwide (Stallones 1980). Major risk factors for ischemic heart disease among New Mexico's non-Hispanic white population parallel U.S. profiles for whites (Samet et al. 1982; New Mexico Health and Environment Department 1987), and the lower ischemic heart disease mortality rates for non-Hispanic whites in the State of New Mexico, compared with rates for whites nationwide, has not been adequately explained.

Our study has several limitations that must be addressed. The limited validity of death certificate cause-of-death statements has been well described for numerous diseases (Engel et al. 1980; Percy, Stanek, and Gloeckler 1981; Kircher, Nelson, and Burdo 1985; Sorlie and Gold 1987), and for cardiovascular disease in particular (Sorlie and Gold 1987). In New Mexico, additional bias in death certificate-based studies may be related to ethnic group. For example, a larger proportion of death certificates was coded under the category "symptoms, signs, and ill-defined conditions" (see Chapter 11) for American Indians than for the other ethnic groups (Samet et al. 1980), suggesting that misclassification of cardiac-related deaths may be greater among American Indians than among non-Indians. Additional bias may enter this study from the changes in the ICD codes for ischemic heart disease (U.S. Department of Health, Education, and Welfare 1979; Sorlic and Gold 1987). However, the adjustments in the classification of ischemic heart disease mortality were designed to reduce artifactual changes in mortality rates caused by inconsistencies in the coding schemes spanning the ICD seventh, eighth, and ninth revisions. Sorlie and Gold observed that, at least for chronic ischemic heart disease in New Mexico, little change in mortality was apparent between the eighth and ninth revision coding schemes (Sorlie and Gold 1987). The adjustment from the ninth to the eighth revision may bias our results toward the null; that is, no recent decline in ischemic heart disease mortality in New Mexico. Nevertheless, our potentially over-adjusted mortality rates still reveal a decline in ischemic heart disease mortality in all ethnic groups during the most recent time period of this study.

Summary

Ischemic heart disease mortality rates in New Mexico were unduly disparate as examined by ethnic and gender group, with highest rates for non-Hispanic white males throughout the 75-year period of these data. Extremely low ischemic heart disease mortality rates were documented for American Indians in New Mexico, while Hispanics generally had rates intermediate between non-Hispanic whites and American Indians. As was observed for whites nationwide, a rise-and-fall pattern of ischemic heart disease mortality was apparent for each of the three major ethnic populations in the state.

These cited data suggest that further investigation of risk factors for ischemic heart disease is warranted, especially among minority peoples of the state.

REFERENCES

Buechley, R. W., C. R. Key, D. L. Morris, W. E. Morton, and M. V. Morgan. 1979. Altitude and ischemic heart disease in tri-cultural New Mexico: an example of confounding. *Am.J.Epidemiol.* 109:663–666.

Coulehan, J. L., G. Lerner, K. Helzlsouer, T. K. Welty, and J. McLaughlin. 1986. Acute myocardial infarction among Navajo Indians, 1976–83. *Am.J.Public Health* 76:412–414.

DeStefano, F., J. L. Coulehan, and M. K. Wiant. 1979. Blood pressure survey on the Navajo Indian Reservation. *Am.J.Epidemiol.* 109:335–345.

Engel, L. W., J. A. Strauchen, L. Chiazze, Jr., and M. Heid. 1980. Accuracy of death certification in an autopsied population with specific attention to malignant neoplasms and vascular diseases. *Am.J.Epidemiol.* 111:99–112.

Franco, L. J., M. P. Stern, M. Rosenthal, S. M. Haffner, H. P. Hazuda, and P. J. Coreaux. 1985. Prevalence, detection, and control of hypertension in a biethnic community. The San Antonio heart study. *Am.J.Epidemiol.* 121:684–696.

Friis, R., G. Nanjundappa, T. J. Prendergast, and M. Welsh. 1981. Coronary heart disease mortality and risk among Hispanics and non-Hispanics in Orange County, California. *Public Health Rep.* 96:418–422.

Gardner, L. I., M. P. Stern, S. M. Haffner, S. P. Gaskill, H. P. Hazuda, J. H. Relethford, and C. W. Eifler. 1984. Prevalence of diabetes in Mexican Americans. Relationship to percent of gene pool derived from Native American sources. *Diabetes* 33:86–92.

Garnick, M. B., P. H. Bennett, and T. Langer, 1979. Low density lipoproteins metabolism and lipoprotein cholesterol content in south-western American Indians. *J.Lipid Res.* 20:31–39.

Gilbert, J. 1955. Absence of coronary thrombosis in Navajo Indians. *Calif.Med.* 82:114–115.

Hanis, C. L., R. E. Ferrell, S. A. Barton, L. Aguilar, A. Garza-Ibarra, B. R. Tulloch, C. A. Garcia, and W. J. Schull. 1983. Diabetes among Mexican Americans in Starr County, Texas. *Am.J.Epidemiol.* 118:659–672.

Kircher, T., J. Nelson, and H. Burdo. 1985. The autopsy as a measure of accuracy of the death certificate. *N.Engl.J.Med.* 313:1263–1269.

Knowler, W. C., D. J. Pettitt, P. J. Savage, and P. H. Bennett. 1981. Diabetes incidence in Pima Indians: contribution of obesity and parental diabetes. *Am.J.Epidemiol.* 113:144–156.

Kraus, B. S. 1954. *The disease picture. Indian health in Arizona.* Chap. VI, p 75. Tucson, AZ: University of Arizona Press.

Kraus, J. F., N. O. Borhani, and C. E. Franti. 1980. Socio-economic status, ethnicity, and risk of coronary heart disease. *Am.J.Epidemiol.* 111:407–414.

Marcus, A. C., and L. A. Crane. 1985. Smoking behavior among U.S. Latinos: an emerging challenge for public health. *Am.J.Public Health* 75:169–172.

Markides, K. S., J. Coreil, and L. A. Ray. 1987. Smoking among Mexican Americans: a three generation study. *Am.J.Public Health* 77:708–711.

Mueller, W. H., S. K. Joos, C. L. Hanis, A. N. Zavaleta, J. Eichner, and W. J. Schull. 1984. The diabetes alert study: growth, fatness, and fat patterning, adolescence through adulthood in Mexican Americans. *Am.J.Phys.Anthropol.* 64:389–399.

New Mexico Health and Environment Department, Office of Health Promotion. 1987. New Mexico behavioral risk factor survey data 1986. Santa Fe, NM.

Office of Technology and Assessment. 1986. *Indian health care.* Washington, DC: U.S. Government Printing Office.

Percy, C., E. Stanek, and L. Gloeckler. 1981. Accuracy of cancer death certificates and its effect on cancer mortality statistics. *Am.J.Public Health* 71:242–250.

Salsbury, C. G. 1937. Disease incidence among Navajos. *Southwest Med.* 21:230–233.

Samet, J. M., C. R. Key, D. M. Kutvirt, and C. L. Wiggins. 1980. Respiratory disease mortality in New Mexico's American Indians and Hispanics. *Am.J. Public Health* 70:492–497.

Samet, J. M., S. D. Schrag, C. A. Howard, C. R. Key, and D. R. Pathak. 1982. Respiratory disease in a New Mexico population sample of Hispanic and non-Hispanic whites. *Am.Rev.Respir.Dis.* 125:152–157.

Samet, J. M., D. B. Coultas, C. A. Howard, B. J. Skipper, and C. L. Hanis. 1988. Diabetes, gallbladder disease, obesity, and hypertension among Hispanics in New Mexico. *Am.J.Epidemiol.* 128:1302–1311.

Schoen, R., and V. E. Nelson. 1981. Mortality by cause among Spanish-surnamed Californians, 1969–1971. *Soc.Sci.Quart.* 62:259–274.

Sievers, M. L. 1966. Disease patterns among southwestern Indians. *Public Health Reports* 81:1075–1083.

———. 1967. Myocardial infarction among southwestern American Indians. *Ann.Intern.Med.* 67:800–807.

———. 1968a. Serum cholesterol levels in southwestern American Indians. *J.Chronic Dis.* 21:107–115.

———. 1968b. Cigarette and alcohol usage by southwestern American Indians. *Am.J.Public Health* 58:71–82.

———. 1976. Diabetes mellitus in American Indians—standard for diagnosis and management. *Diabetes* 25:528–531.

———. 1977. Historical overview of hypertension among American Indians and Alaskan Natives. *Ariz.Med.* 34:607–610.

Sievers, M. L., and J. R. Fisher. 1979. Increasing rate of acute myocardial infarction in Southwestern American Indians. *Ariz.Med.* 36:739.

Smith, R. L., C. G. Salsbury, and A. G. Gilliam. 1956. Recorded and expected mortality among the Navajo with special reference to cancer. *J.Natl.Cancer Inst.* 17:77–89.

Sorlie, P. D., and E. B. Gold. 1987. The effect of physician terminology preference on coronary heart disease mortality: an artifact uncovered by the ninth revision ICD. *Am.J.Public Health* 77:148–152.

Stallones, R. A. 1980. The rise and fall of ischemic heart disease. *Sci.Am.* 243:53–59.

Stern, M. P., and S. P. Gaskill. 1978. Secular trends in ischemic heart disease and stroke mortality from 1970 to 1976 in Spanish surnamed and other white individuals in Bexar County, Texas. *Circulation* 58:537–543.

Stern, M. P., J. A. Pugh, S. P. Gaskill, and H. P. Hazuda. 1982a. Knowledge, attitudes, and behavior related to obesity and dieting in Mexican Americans and Anglos: the San Antonio heart study. *Am.J.Epidemiol.* 115:917–928.

Stern, M. P., S. P. Gaskill, C. R. Allen, V. Garza, J. L. Gonzales, and R. H. Waldrop. 1982b. Cardiovascular risk factors in Mexican Americans in Laredo, Texas. II. Prevalence and control of hypertension. *Am.J.Epidemiol.* 113:556–562.

Stern, M. P., M. Rosenthal, S. M. Haffner, H. P. Hazuda, and L. J. Franco. 1984. Sex difference in the effects of socio-cultural status on diabetes and cardiovascular risk factors in Mexican Americans. *Am.J.Epidemiol.* 120:834–851.

Stern, M. P., S. P. Gaskill, C. R. Allen, V. Garza, J. L. Gonzales, and R. H. Waldrop. 1985. Cardiovascular risk factors in Mexican Americans in Laredo, Texas. I. Prevalence of overweight and diabetes and distribution of serum lipids. *Am.J.Epidemiol.* 113:546–555.

Stern, M. P., B. S. Bradshaw, C. W. Eifler, D. S. Fong, H. P. Hazuda, and M. Rosenthal. 1987. Secular decline in death rates due to ischemic heart disease in Mexican Americans and non-Hispanic whites in Texas, 1970–1980. *Circulation* 76:1245–1250.

Stern, M. P., S. M. Haffner, H. P. Hazuda, and M. Rosenthal. In press. Cardiovascular disease in Mexican Americans. (Chapter.) In *Woodlands Proceedings of the Conference on Health of the Hispanic Population*, edited by C. Hanis and M. K. Stern.

U.S. Department of Health, Education, and Welfare. 1979. *Proceedings of the*

Conference on the Decline in Coronary Heart Disease Mortality. Washington, DC: U.S. Government Printing Office.
U.S. Department of Health and Human Services. 1983. *Cardiovascular disease: a report of the Surgeon General.* Washington, DC: U.S. Government Printing Office.
West, K. M. 1974. Diabetes in American Indians and other native populations of the New World. *Diabetes* 23:841–855.
———. 1978. Diabetes in American Indians. *Adv.Metab.Dis.* 9:29–48.
World Health Organization. 1957. *Manual of the International Statistical Classification of Diseases, Injuries, and Causes of Death.* Based on the recommendations of the Seventh Revision Conference, 1955. Geneva, Switzerland: WHO.
———. 1967. *Manual of the International Statistical Classification of Diseases, Injuries, and Causes of Death.* Based on the recommendations of the Eighth Revision Conference, 1965. Geneva, Switzerland: WHO.
———. 1977. *Manual of the International Statistical Classification of Diseases, Injuries, and Causes of Death.* Based on the recommendations of the Ninth Revision Conference, 1975. Geneva, Switzerland: WHO.

CHAPTER 7

Respiratory Disease Mortality

Jonathan M. Samet

Mortality rates for two of the major lung diseases, lung cancer and chronic obstructive pulmonary disease, have been shown to vary among different racial and ethnic groups in the United States. Both of these diseases have been closely linked to cigarette smoking. Since the 1950's, descriptive studies have documented differing patterns of these two cigarette-related diseases in Hispanic and non-Hispanic whites in the West and Southwest. In California during the 1950's and 1960's, mortality rates from lung cancer among older Mexican-born females were two to three times the rates for all California women (Buechley et al. 1957; Buell, Mendez, and Dunn 1968). Mortality data from Texas (Lee, Roberts, and Darwin 1976) and from New Mexico (Samet et al. 1980) have shown a similar pattern of ethnic differences in women. In New Mexico and Texas (Samet et al. 1980), California (Menck et al. 1975), and Colorado (Berg 1980), mortality and incidence rates for lung cancer have been substantially lower for Hispanic males than for non-Hispanic white males. Similar observations have been made in New Mexico for chronic obstructive pulmonary disease (Samet et al. 1980). Lower cigarette smoking by Hispanic than by non-Hispanic whites has been documented in cross-sectional surveys in the West and Southwest (Samet et al. 1982; Marcus and Crane 1985) and nationwide (Remington et al. 1985; National Center for Health Statistics 1986). However, longitudinal data on smoking and smoking-related diseases among Hispanics and other minority populations are scant (Baquet et al. 1986; Savitz 1986).

Rates of cigarette-related respiratory diseases also differ between southwestern American Indians and non-Hispanic whites. Both mortality and incidence data show that lung cancer is infrequent among American Indians (Smith, Salsbury, and Gillian 1956; Sievers and Cohen 1961; Samet et al. 1980). Mortality data for New Mexico demonstrate that chronic obstructive pulmonary disease is also an infrequent cause of death in American Indians. Limited evidence suggests that few American Indians in the Southwest regularly smoke cigarettes (DeStefano, Coulehan, and Wiant 1979; Sievers 1968; Samet et al. 1984).

New Mexico's large populations of American Indians and Hispanics provide an opportunity to describe disease occurrence in these minority groups. To further characterize cigarette-related diseases in Hispanics and in American Indians, we examined mortality from lung cancer and from chronic obstructive pulmonary disease in New Mexico for the period 1958 through 1982 by racial and ethnic group.

Methodologic Considerations

Cause of death was coded according to the seventh, eighth, and ninth revisions of the International Classification of Diseases (ICD) (World Health Organization 1957, 1967, 1977). Deaths were assigned to chronic obstructive pulmonary disease if they were due to chronic bronchitis (ICD7 502, ICD8 and ICD9 491), to emphysema (ICD7 527.1, ICD8 and ICD9 492), to chronic obstructive lung disease (ICD8 519.3), or to chronic obstructive pulmonary disease (ICD9 496). We also examined mortality from cancers of the lung, trachea, and bronchus (ICD7 162.0–162.1, 162.8–163, ICD8 and ICD9 162).

Results

During the period 1958 through 1982, age-adjusted mortality from lung cancer and from chronic obstructive pulmonary disease increased progressively in Hispanic and non-Hispanic white males (Table 7.1). Across the study period, mortality rates for lung cancer in non-Hispanic whites were lower in New Mexico than in the U.S. in general, whereas mortality rates for chronic obstructive pulmonary disease were much higher. For all time periods, however, the rates for these diseases were substantially lower in Hispanics than in non-Hispanic whites. For American Indians, rates were even lower in all time periods, and clear temporal trends were not present.

Age-specific mortality rates for lung cancer were examined by birth cohort for Hispanics and non-Hispanic whites (Figures 7.1 through 7.4). In non-Hispanic white males, mortality rates increased progressively only at older ages for successive birth cohorts, but were stable or declined in more recent birth cohorts at younger ages. Age-specific rates for Hispanic males were lower at all ages for these diseases. For lung cancer in Hispanic males, the age-specific mortality rates rose for each successive birth cohort. For chronic obstructive pulmonary disease, similar temporal trends were evident only for the three oldest age groups, but numbers of deaths were small in the younger age groups (data not shown).

In women, mortality from lung cancer and from chronic obstructive

Table 7.1
Mortality rates* in New Mexican males and U.S. white males from lung cancer and chronic obstructive pulmonary disease (COPD), 1958 through 1982

	Time period (inclusive years)				
	1958–62	1963–67	1968–72	1973–77	1978–82
Lung cancer					
Non-Hispanic white	30.1	34.6	48.3	56.6	62.9
Hispanic	10.1	14.5	18.2	20.1	28.8
American Indian	5.3	4.7	9.0	7.7	10.8
U.S. white	38.5	47.5	57.8	64.8	70.4
COPD					
Non-Hispanic white	17.0	41.8	48.0	56.3	64.5
Hispanic	5.0	11.4	13.0	20.6	30.1
American Indian	1.4	8.0	4.2	13.9	12.2
U.S. white	13.7	24.8	31.4	35.1	37.3

Source: Adapted from Samet et al. 1988b, printed with permission.
* Age-adjusted annual rates per 100,000.

pulmonary disease also increased in both Hispanic and non-Hispanic whites from 1958 through 1982 (Table 7.2). The rate of increase, however, was much greater for the non-Hispanic white women. Rates for both diseases were low in American Indian women and varied inconsistently across the study period.

For lung cancer in non-Hispanic white women, age-specific rates increased with successive birth cohorts at older ages (Figure 7.2). Similarly, age-specific rates for chronic obstructive pulmonary disease increased for successive birth cohorts at all ages (data not shown). Lung cancer mortality leveled for the more recently born Hispanic women at older ages (Figure 7.4), but this pattern was less consistent for chronic obstructive pulmonary disease (data not shown). Consistent temporal trends were not evident at younger ages.

Discussion

These longitudinal observations on mortality in New Mexico confirm other studies of the differing patterns of occurrence of the major cigarette-related respiratory diseases in American Indians, Hispanic whites,

LUNG CANCER MORTALITY
NON-HISPANIC WHITE MALES

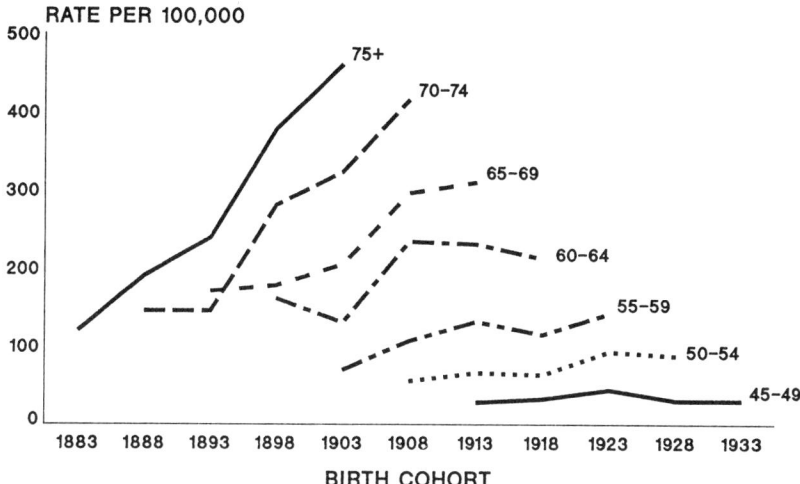

Figure 7.1. *Lung cancer mortality in non-Hispanic white males in New Mexico, by 5-year birth cohort.*
Source: Samet *et al.* 1988b, printed with permission

and non-Hispanics. The contrasts among these populations are sharp and cannot be explained by problems related to calculation of the ethnic-specific rates or to errors in the assignment of cause of death.

The validity of death certificate cause-of-death statements for lung cancer and for chronic obstructive pulmonary disease has been described in other populations (Mitchell *et al.* 1968; Percy, Stanek, and Gloeckler 1981). In New Mexico, possible bias related to ethnic group in assigning cause of death is plausible. Clinicians may fail to diagnose lung cancer and chronic obstructive pulmonary disease in American Indians and Hispanics because they are aware of the descriptive epidemiology of these diseases in New Mexico. We also found substantial differences among the three ethnic groups in the extent to which deaths were attributed to the category of symptoms, signs, and ill-defined conditions (see chapter 11).

Previous studies in New Mexico have documented the lesser occurrence of lung cancer and chronic obstructive pulmonary disease in Hispanic males than in non-Hispanic white males (Samet 1980, 1982), and

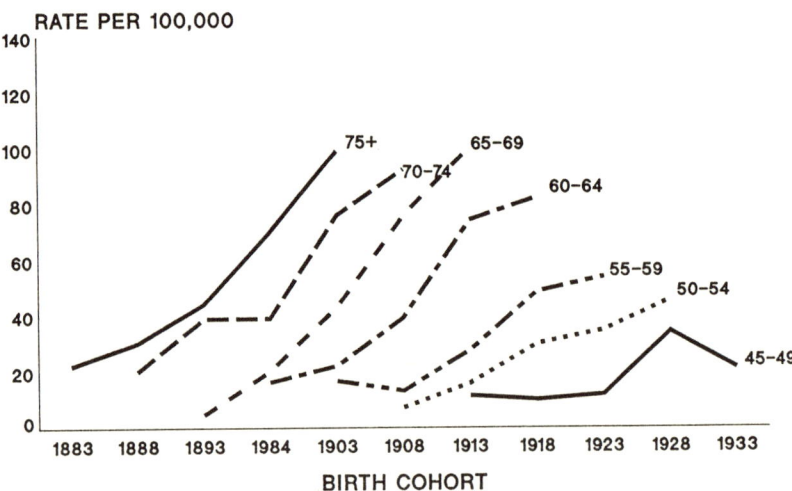

Figure 7.2. *Lung cancer mortality in non-Hispanic white females in New Mexico, by 5-year birth cohort.*
Source: Samet *et al.* 1988b, printed with permission

the greater mortality from chronic obstructive pulmonary disease in non-Hispanic white males than in U.S. whites (Samet 1980). The higher mortality from chronic obstructive pulmonary disease in non-Hispanic white males probably reflects migration of affected persons to the Southwest (Lebowitz and Burrows 1975). Based on a respiratory disease survey conducted in 1978 and 1979 and a lung cancer case-control study conducted from 1980 through 1982, we have explained the lesser occurrence of these diseases in Hispanic males by the lower daily consumption of cigarettes by Hispanic male smokers. However, data from a 1984 to 1985 population survey conducted in Hispanic residents of a New Mexico community suggested increasing cigarette consumption by young adult and middle-aged males (Samet *et al.* 1988a). The strong trends of increasing mortality from lung cancer and from chronic obstructive pulmonary disease across the study period also imply increasing smoking by Hispanic males. A similar increase in lung cancer has been described for Spanish-surname males in the Denver area across the periods bounded by 1969 through 1971 and 1979 through 1981 (Savitz 1986).

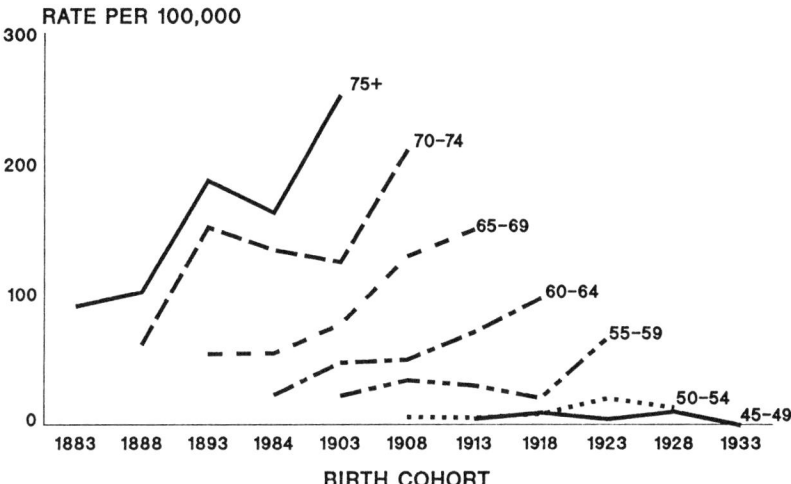

Figure 7.3. *Lung cancer mortality in Hispanic males in New Mexico, by 5-year birth cohort.*
Source: Samet *et al.* 1988b, printed with permission

In New Mexico and other states, older Hispanic women have had particularly high mortality from lung cancer (Buechley *et al.* 1957; Buell, Mendez, and Dunn 1968; Lee, Roberts, and Darwin 1976; Samet *et al.* 1980), a pattern attributed to the smoking of hand-rolled cigarettes (Buell, Mendez, and Dunn 1968; Humble *et al.* 1985). In New Mexico, lung cancer mortality has declined in the more-recently born Hispanic women reaching age 70 years and above; this decline is consistent with the cohort effect postulated by Buell and colleagues (Buell, Mendez, and Dunn 1968).

The continued low mortality from cigarette-related diseases in American Indians, and the mortality increases among Hispanics pose challenges for those concerned with the health of these minority groups. The tobacco industry has targeted advertising toward the Hispanic population of the U.S. (Davis 1987), and success of such advertising will accelerate the trends through 1982 that we have documented. In fact, cigarette smoking is equally prevalent at present among Hispanic and non-Hispanic

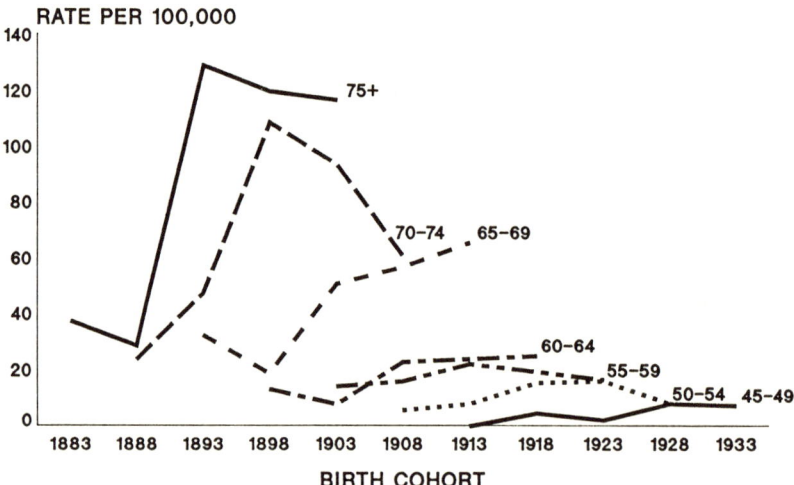

Figure 7.4. *Lung cancer mortality in Hispanic females in New Mexico, by 5-year birth cohort.*
Source: Samet *et al*. 1988b, printed with permission

white schoolchildren in Albuquerque, New Mexico (Greenberg *et al.* 1987). For American Indians in the Southwest, the goal of health education must be to maintain the low prevalence of smoking.

Summary

Our data show that among non-Hispanic whites, age-adjusted mortality rates from lung cancer and from chronic obstructive pulmonary disease increased progressively in both males and females from 1958 through 1982. Mortality rates for both diseases also increased in Hispanics during the study period, but the most recent rates for Hispanics were well below those for other non-Hispanic whites. Age-specific mortality rates for lung cancer declined for more-recently born Hispanic women at older ages. In American Indians, rates for both diseases were low throughout the study period and did not show consistent temporal trends.

Table 7.2
Mortality rates* in New Mexican females and U.S. white females from lung cancer and chronic obstructive pulmonary disease (COPD), 1958 through 1982

	Time period (inclusive years)				
	1958–62	1963–67	1968–72	1973–77	1978–82
Lung cancer					
Non-Hispanic white	4.5	6.8	10.8	17.9	19.9
Hispanic	4.8	5.3	12.7	12.7	11.2
American Indian	1.6	1.9	5.6	2.3	4.2
U.S. white	5.6	7.5	11.1	15.5	21.1
COPD					
Non-Hispanic white	1.6	4.6	7.8	12.9	22.9
Hispanic	2.9	6.2	8.2	12.8	13.7
American Indian	1.7	2.3	0.3	6.7	0.8
U.S. white	2.2	3.7	5.4	7.6	10.9

Source: Adapted from Samet *et al.* 1988b, printed with permission.
* Age-adjusted annual rates per 100,000.

REFERENCES

Baquet, C. R., K. Ringen, E. S. Pollack, J. L. Young, J. W. Horm, L. A. Gloeckler-Ries, and N. K. Simpson. March 1986. *Cancer among blacks and other minorities: statistical profiles.* NIH Publication No. 86–2785. Bethesda, MD: National Cancer Institute.

Berg, J. W. 1980. The real cancer risks in Colorado. *Colo.Med.* 77:241–245.

Buechley, R. W., J. E. Dunn, G. Linden, and L. Breslow. 1957. Excess lung cancer mortality rates among Mexican women in California. *Cancer* 10:63–66.

Buell, P. E., W. M. Mendez, and J. E. Dunn. 1968. Cancer of the lung among Mexican immigrant women in California. *Cancer* 22:186–192.

Davis, R. M. 1987. Current trends in cigarette advertising and marketing. *N.Engl.J.Med.* 316:725–732.

DeStefano, F., J. L. Coulehan, and M. K. Wiant. 1979. Blood pressure survey on the Navajo Indian Reservation. *Am.J.Epidemiol.* 109:335–345.

Greenberg, M. A., C. L. Wiggins, D. M. Kutvirt, and J. M. Samet. 1987. Cigarette use among Hispanic and non-Hispanic white school children, Albuquerque, New Mexico. *Am.J.Public Health* 77:621–622.

Humble, C. G., J. M. Samet, D. R. Pathak, and B. J. Skipper. 1985. Cigarette smoking and lung cancer in "Hispanic" whites and other whites in New Mexico. *Am.J.Public Health* 75:145–148.

Lebowitz, M. D., and B. Burrows. 1975. Tucson epidemiology study of obstructive lung diseases. II: Effects of in-migration factors on the prevalence of obstructive lung disease. *Am.J.Epidemiol.* 102:153–163.

Lee, E. S., R. E. Roberts, and L. R. Darwin. 1976. Excess and deficit lung cancer mortality in three ethnic groups in Texas. *Cancer* 38:2551–2556.

Marcus, A. C., and L. A. Crane. 1985. Smoking behavior among U.S. Latinos: an emerging challenge for public health (commentary). *Am.J.Public Health* 75:169–172.

Menck, H. R., B. E. Henderson, M. C. Pike, T. Mack, S. P. Martin, and J. Soo Hoo. 1975. Cancer incidence in the Mexican American. *J.Natl.Cancer Inst.* 55:531–536.

Mitchell, R. S., G. W. Silvers, G. A. Dart, T. L. Petty, T. N. Vincent, S. F. Ryan, and G. F. Filley. 1968. Clinical and morphologic correlations in chronic airway obstruction. *Am.Rev.Repir.Dis.* 97:54–63.

National Center for Health Statistics. June 30, 1986. C. A. Schoenborn, and B. H. Cohen, eds. *Trends in smoking, alcohol consumption, and other health practices among U.S. adults in 1977 and 1983.* Advance data from Vital and Health Statistics, No. 118. DHHS Publication No. (PHS) 86–1250. Hyattsville, MD: Public Health Service.

Percy, C., E. Stanek, and L. Gloeckler. 1981. Accuracy of cancer death certificates and its effect on cancer mortality statistics. *Am.J.Public Health* 71:242–250.

Remington, P. L., M. R. Forman, E. M. Gentry, J. S. Marks, G. C. Hogelin, and F. L. Trowbridge. 1985. Current smoking trends in the United States. The 1981–1983 behavioral risk factor surveys. *JAMA* 253:2975–2978.

Samet, J. M., C. R. Key, D. M. Kutvirt, and C. L. Wiggins. 1980. Respiratory disease mortality in New Mexico's American Indians and Hispanics. *Am.J. Public Health* 70:492–497.

Samet, J. M., S. D. Schrag, C. A. Howard, C. R. Key, and D. R. Pathak. 1982. Respiratory disease in a New Mexico population sample of Hispanic and non-Hispanic whites. *Am.Rev.Respir.Dis.* 125:152–157.

Samet. J. M., D. M. Kutvirt, R. J. Waxweiler, and C. R. Key. 1984. Uranium mining and lung cancer in Navajo men. *N.Engl.J.Med.* 310:1481–1484.

Samet, J. M., D. B. Coultas, C. A. Howard, and B. J. Skipper. 1988a. Respiratory diseases and cigarette smoking in an Hispanic population in New Mexico. *Am.Rev.Respir.Dis.* 137:814–819.

Samet, J. M., C. L. Wiggins, C. R. Key, and T. M. Becker. 1988b. Mortality from lung disease and chronic obstructive pulmonary disease in New Mexico, 1958–82. *Am.J.Public Health* 78:1182–1186.

Savitz, D. A. 1986. Changes in Spanish surname cancer rates relative to other whites, Denver area, 1969–71 to 1979–81. *Am.J.Public Health* 76:1210–1215.

Sievers, M. L. 1968. Cigarette and alcohol usage by southwestern American Indians. *Am.J.Public Health* 58:71–82.

Sievers, M. L., and S. L. Cohen. 1961. Lung cancer among Indians of the southwestern United States. *Ann.Intern.Med.* 54:912–915.

Smith, R. L., C. G. Salsbury, and A. G. Gillian. 1956. Recorded and expected mortality among the Navajo, with special reference to cancer. *J.Natl.Cancer Inst.* 17:77–89.

World Health Organization. 1957. *Manual of the International Statistical Classifiction of Diseases, Injuries, and Causes of Death*. Based on the recommendations of the Seventh Revision Conference, 1955. Geneva, Switzerland: WHO.

——— 1967. *Manual of the International Statistical Classification of Diseases, Injuries, and Causes of Death*. Based on the recommendations of the Eighth Revision Conference, 1965. Geneva, Switzerland: WHO.

——— 1977. *Manual of the International Statistical Classification of Diseases, Injuries, and Causes of Death*. Based on the recommendations of the Ninth Revision Conference, 1975. Geneva, Switzerland: WHO.

CHAPTER 8

Alcohol-Related Mortality

Liza D. Chavez
Thomas M. Becker
Charles L. Wiggins
Charles R. Key
Jonathan M. Samet

Alcohol-related illness is a major cause of morbidity and mortality in the U.S., where in recent years over 26,000 deaths each year have been directly related to alcohol (Centers for Disease Control [CDC] 1989). The ninth leading cause of death in the U.S. is cirrhosis of the liver (CDC 1989), a disease frequently caused by chronic alcohol abuse. Alcoholism in the U.S. creates a heavy health and economic burden that is not distributed uniformly among the various ethnic groups in the nation.

National data indicate that rates of alcohol-related morbidity and mortality in the U.S. are higher among blacks (CDC 1989) and American Indians (May 1986) than among whites. Published data also indicate high rates for Hispanics in the U.S., although the number of published studies on Hispanic alcoholism and alcohol-related morbidity and mortality is small despite the fact that Hispanics constitute the second largest minority group in the U.S. (U.S. Bureau of the Census 1981). The reports on Hispanics are also limited by their small study populations, which are confined mainly to Hispanics living in Texas and California.

In this chapter we examine trends in alcohol-related mortality in the three major ethnic groups of New Mexico. Our analyses provide baseline information on alcohol-related mortality among these ethnic groups from a population-based perspective over a 25-year period from 1958 through 1982.

Methodologic Considerations

For this report, deaths attributed to alcohol included International Classification of Diseases (ICD) codes listed in Table 8.1. Numbers of deaths

Table 8.1
Alcohol-related categories, and corresponding codes in the seventh, eighth, and ninth revisions of the International Classification of Diseases

Category	ICD7	ICD8	ICD9
Alcoholic psychosis	307	291	291.0–291.9
Alcoholism*	322	303	303, 305.0, 425.5, 357.5, 535.3
Chronic alcoholic liver disease	581.1	571.1	571.0–571.3
Other specified and unspecified chronic liver disease	581.0, 582, 583	571.8, 571.9	571.4, 571.5, 571.6, 571.8, 571.9, 572.3

*Includes alcoholic cardiomyopathy, alcoholic polyneuropathy, alcoholic gastritis, and nondependent abuse of alcohol.

were not adjusted to one ICD coding scheme over the 25-year study period because of high comparability ratios for coding of alcohol-related mortality among the three ICD revisions (CDC 1984).

Results

Alcohol-related mortality rates throughout the 25-year study period varied markedly by ethnic group in New Mexico (Table 8.2). For both sexes, American Indians consistently had a higher age-adjusted rate than did Hispanics or non-Hispanic whites for each 5-year period; rates for Hispanic males far exceeded rates for non-Hispanic white males, although rates for females in the two groups were comparable. For all three ethnic groups in all time periods, age-adjusted alcohol-related mortality rates for males exceeded those for females, with the rate difference within each ethnic group generally at least twofold higher for males than for females. The data show increasing alcohol-related mortality by time period, with extremely high rates for American Indian males from 1973 through 1977 (197.8 per 100,000 persons).

Examination of the data by 5-year birth cohorts from 1883 through 1928 reveals markedly different patterns among the ethnic groups (Fig-

Table 8.2
Alcohol-related mortality rates* in New Mexicans by ethnic group and sex, 1958 through 1982

	Time period (inclusive years)				
	1958–62	1963–67	1968–72	1973–77	1978–82
Males					
Non-Hispanic white	17.0	19.0	18.8	24.4	25.5
Hispanic	25.3	33.4	54.0	63.9	64.8
American Indian	28.5	32.8	108.0	197.8	119.1
Females					
Non-Hispanic white	9.0	9.8	9.7	12.0	10.4
Hispanic	9.7	11.2	14.0	11.0	16.1
American Indian	18.6	26.7	53.0	68.7	38.3

* Age-adjusted rates per 100,000, adjusted to 1970 U.S. population.

ures 8.1 through 8.6). A sharp rise-and-fall pattern of alcohol-related mortality among American Indian men and women is apparent for all age groups (Figures 8.5 and 8.6). However, for Hispanic males, age-specific alcohol-related mortality increased in most age groups (Figure 8.3). The patterns observed for Hispanic and non-Hispanic white women and for non-Hispanic white males are similar—alcohol-related mortality rates decreased slightly, leveled off, and then again increased (Figures 8.1, 8.2, 8.4).

Discussion

Our data for New Mexico clearly show striking differences in the alcohol-related mortality rates among American Indians, Hispanics, and non-Hispanic whites. American Indians are shown to be at highest risk of death from alcohol-related illness, followed by Hispanics and then non-Hispanic whites. The risk has increased since 1958 for all three ethnic groups.

Numerous studies conducted nationwide among American Indians have reported high alcohol-related mortality rates (Kunitz *et al.* 1971; Carr and Lee 1977; Westermeyer and Peake 1983). Our analyses reaffirm these findings, and show that American Indians in New Mexico are also at high risk of death from alcohol-related illness. In Indian Health Service Areas throughout the U.S., alcohol-related mortality consistently exceeds

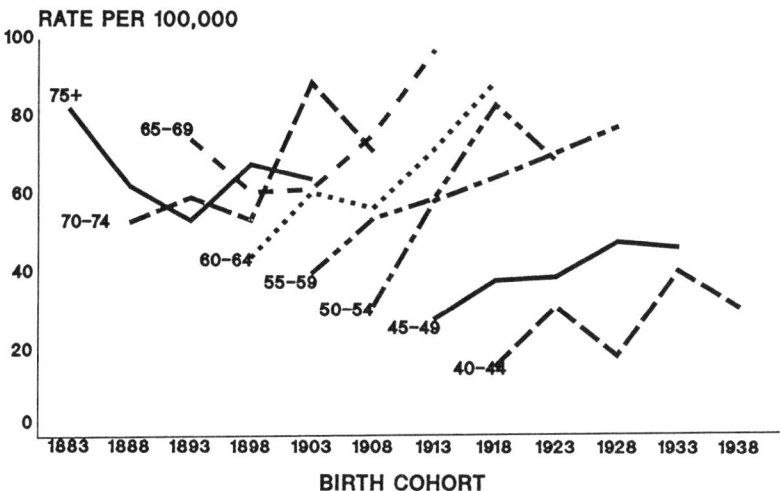

Figure 8.1. *Alcohol-related mortality among non-Hispanic white males in New Mexico, by 5-year birth cohort.*

rates for all other races in the U.S. (U.S. Department of Health and Human Services 1988). In the Southwest, a study of liver cirrhosis death rates among Hopi Indians of Arizona found the rates to be more than four times the rate for the general U.S. population (Kunitz et al. 1971). The extent of alcoholism among the Navajo population is unknown; however, death rates from alcoholism among Navajo Indians were 5.5 times higher than rates for the overall U.S. population (May 1986), and Navajo tribal officials recognize alcoholism as the tribe's number one problem (Ferguson 1970).

For Hispanics, the few published studies that have examined alcohol-related deaths have shown either high rates or increasing rates in this ethnic group. An autopsy series reported from the University of Southern California Medical Center in Los Angeles County showed that alcohol-related deaths among Hispanics rose from 4% of all autopsies in 1950 to 18% in 1970 (Edmondson 1975). In San Antonio, Texas, Hispanics had a cirrhosis death rate in 1980 of 11 per 100,000 population as compared with a rate of 9.7 per 100,000 for Anglos (Caetano 1983). However, in

ALCOHOL-RELATED MORTALITY
NON-HISPANIC WHITE FEMALES

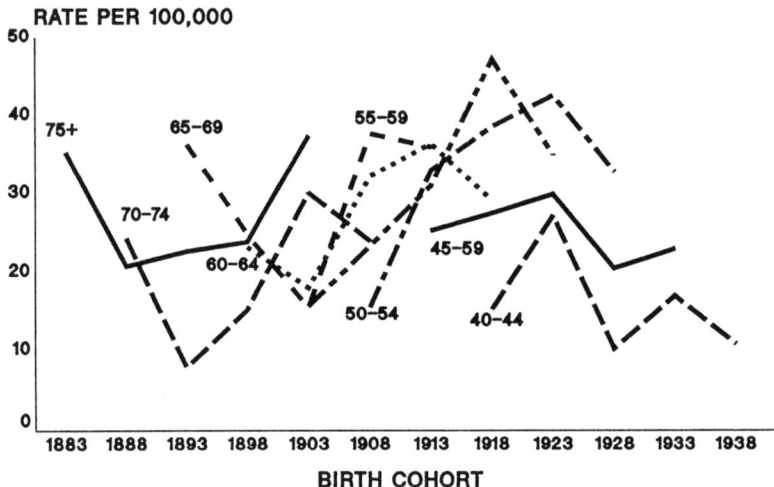

Figure 8.2. *Alcohol-related mortality among non-Hispanic white females in New Mexico, by 5-year birth cohort.*

Cook County, Mexico-born Hispanics showed a lower death rate from cirrhosis than did whites, while Puerto Rico-born Hispanics showed a higher death rate than did whites for the years 1979 through 1981 (Shai and Rosenwaike 1987). Clearly, it is not possible to make sweeping generalizations about Hispanics in reference to alcohol-related mortality. It has been suggested, however, that high death rates from alcoholism among some groups of Hispanics may reflect a more accepting social attitude toward intoxication than that held by non-Hispanic whites (Caetano 1984).

Racial differences in alcohol tolerance have been hypothesized to cause the high rates of alcohol abuse and alcohol-related mortality among American Indians; however, Bennion and Li (1976) found that mean rates of alcohol metabolism were almost identical between American Indians and whites. In addition, researchers from this study reported no racial differences in hepatic alcohol dehydrogenase activity and isoenzyme pattern in liver biopsy specimens.

Although the alcohol-related mortality rates reported in New Mexico

ALCOHOL-RELATED MORTALITY
HISPANIC MALES

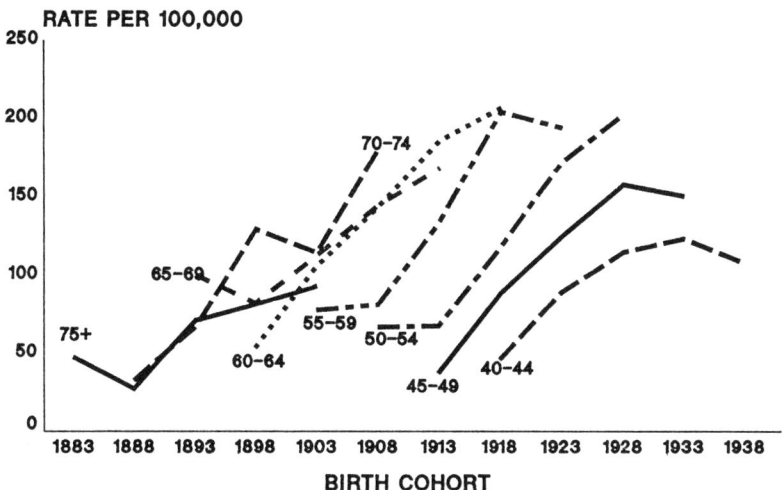

Figure 8.3. *Alcohol-related mortality among Hispanic males in New Mexico, by 5-year birth cohort.*

are high, the rates underestimate the actual risk. For this study, the definition of alcohol-related mortality included only deaths that could be completely attributed to alcohol use, such as alcoholism, alcoholic cirrhosis of the liver, alcoholic psychosis, alcoholic cardiomyopathy, alcoholic polyneuropathy, alcoholic gastritis, and nondependent abuse of alcohol. This list excludes other categories of deaths that may have been alcohol related, such as deaths from unintentional injuries, suicides, and homicides. Alcohol involvement also plays a significant role in fatal motor vehicle accidents, and New Mexico ranks highest in motor vehicle accident fatalities in the U.S. (New Mexico Highway and Transportation Department 1989a). In 51% of the deaths from traffic crashes in 1986, decedents' blood alcohol levels were present (New Mexico Highway and Transportation Department 1989b). A large proportion of pedestrian fatalities in the state also are connected with high blood alcohol levels. Alcohol was present in 49% of homicide victims and in 42% of the suicides in New Mexico in 1985 (New Mexico Office of the Medical Investigator 1985). Since approximately half of the fatal injuries in New Mex-

ALCOHOL-RELATED MORTALITY
HISPANIC FEMALES

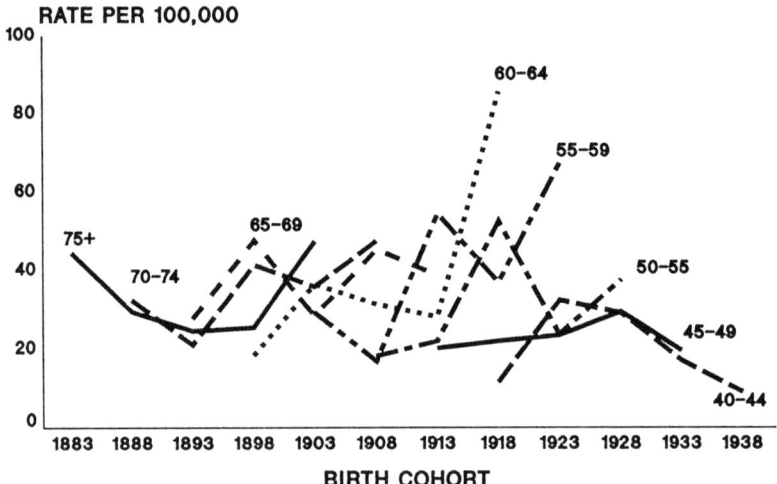

Figure 8.4. *Alcohol-related mortality among Hispanic females in New Mexico, by 5-year birth cohort.*

ico are associated with alcohol consumption, the data presented in this study, which do not include such deaths, can be considered to give only minimum estimates of the alcohol-related mortality rates.

Numbers of reported alcohol-related mortality rates are also subject to bias from underreporting by physicians, who frequently fail to report alcohol misuse as the underlying cause of death on a death certificate. Cirrhosis, for example, can be completely asymptomatic and clinically impossible to detect; and in such a case, the lack of correlation between clinical symptoms and underlying disease will probably lead to misclassification of the underlying cause of death (Blake *et al.* 1988). In over 40% of subjects with biopsy-proven alcoholic cirrhosis, the death certificate contained no reference to either alcohol abuse or liver disease (Blake *et al.* 1988). In a study assessing the validity of death certificate data for alcohol-related mortality among U.S. Army veterans, a review of medical records revealed more than six times the number of alcohol-related deaths shown in the death certificates (Pollock *et al.* 1987).

Other potential sources of bias in our data set are discussed in various

ALCOHOL-RELATED MORTALITY
AMERICAN INDIAN MALES

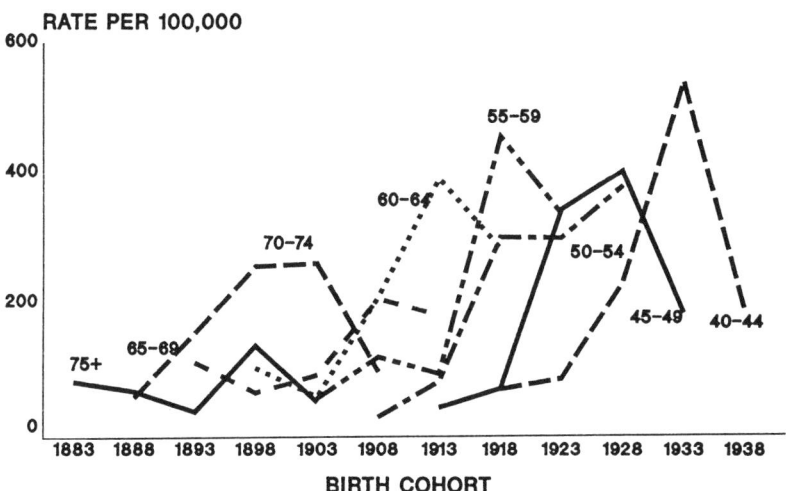

Figure 8.5. *Alcohol-related mortality among American Indian males in New Mexico, by 5-year birth cohort.*

chapters of this book. These other sources include ethnic misclassification, and deaths being registered as occurring from symptoms, signs, and ill-defined conditions. Despite these potential sources of bias, our data show the alcohol-related mortality rates to be extremely high in the minority populations of New Mexico—especially among men—when compared with rates in the white majority in the state.

Summary

Alcohol-related illness is a major cause of mortality in New Mexico, a state that ranks second in the nation in alcohol-related mortality rates. For both sexes, the data show that American Indians consistently had higher alcohol-related mortality rates than did Hispanics or non-Hispanic whites from 1958 through 1982. Mortality rates for Hispanic men far exceeded rates for non-Hispanic white men; however, Hispanic mortality rates among women were comparable to rates for non-Hispanic white women. The data also showed increasing mortality from alcohol over the study

ALCOHOL-RELATED MORTALITY
AMERICAN INDIAN FEMALES

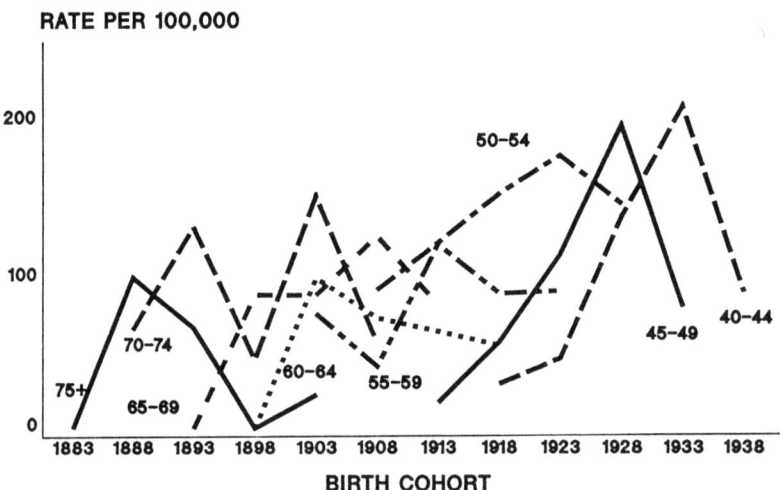

Figure 8.6.   *Alcohol-related mortality among American Indian females in New Mexico, by 5-year birth cohort.*

period, with the highest rates among American Indian men from 1973 through 1977 (197.8 per 100,000). Considering that many fatal injuries in New Mexico are related to alcohol consumption, we suggest that the results of our data are only a minimum estimate of the extremely high alcohol-related mortality rates in this state.

REFERENCES

Bennion, L. J., and T. K. Li. 1976. Alcohol metabolism in American Indians and whites: lack of racial differences in metabolic rate and liver alcohol dehydrogenase. *N.Engl.J.Med.* 294:9–13.

Blake, J. E., K. V. Compton, W. Schmidt, D. Jur, and H. Orrego. 1988. Accuracy of death certificates in the diagnosis of alcoholic liver cirrhosis. *Alcoholism (NY)* 12:168–171.

Caetano, R. 1983. Drinking patterns and alcohol problems among Hispanics in the U.S.: a review. *Drug Alcohol Depend.* 12:37–59.

———. 1984. Ethnicity and drinking in northern California: a comparison among whites, blacks, and Hispanics. *Alcohol Alcohol* 19:31–44.

Carr, B. A., and E. S. Lee. 1977. Navajo tribal mortality: a life table analysis of the leading causes of death. *Soc.Biol.* 25:279–287.

Centers for Disease Control. 1984. A system to convert ICD diagnostic codes for alcohol research. *Morbidity and Mortality Weekly Reports* 33:216–223.

———. 1989. Alcohol-related deaths—United States, 1968–1978. *Morbidity and Mortality Weekly Reports* 38:649–651.

Edmondson, H. A. 1975. *Mexican-American alcoholism and deaths at LAC-USC Medical Center.* Testimony before Subcommittee on Alcoholism of the California Senate.

Ferguson, F. N. 1970. A treatment program for Navajo alcoholics. Results after 4 years. *J.Stud.Alcohol* 31:898–919.

Kunitz, S. J., J. E. Levy, C. L. Odoroff, and J. Bollinger. 1971. The epidemiology of alcoholic cirrhosis in two southwestern Indian tribes. *J.Stud.Alcohol* 32:706–720.

May, P. A. 1986. Alcohol and drug misuse prevention programs for American Indians: needs and opportunities. *J.Stud.Alcohol* 47:187–195.

New Mexico Highway and Transportation Department. 1989a. New Mexico traffic accident data 1986. Transportation Program Division, Traffic Safety Bureau, Santa Fe, NM.

———. 1989b. New Mexico traffic crash data 1986. Transportation Program Division, Traffic Safety Bureau, Santa Fe, NM.

New Mexico Office of the Medical Investigator. 1985. *Annual report 1985.* Santa Fe, NM.

Pollock, D. A., C. A. Boyle, F. DeStefano, L. A. Moyer, and M. A. Kirk. 1987. Underreporting of alcohol-related mortality in death certificates of young U.S. Army veterans. *JAMA* 258:345–348.

Shai, D., and I. Rosenwaike. 1987. Mortality among Hispanics in metropolitan Chicago: an examination based on vital statistics data. *J.Chronic Dis.* 40:445–451.

U.S. Bureau of the Census. 1981. *Census of the population, 1980. General population characteristics. Final report.* Washington, DC: U.S. Government Printing Office.

U.S. Department of Health and Human Services. 1988. *Indian Health Service Chart Series Book, April, 1988.* Publication No. 0–218–547:QL3. Washington, DC: U.S. Government Printing Office.

Westermeyer, J., and E. Peake. 1983. Ten-year follow-up of alcoholic Native Americans in Minnesota. *Am.J.Psychiatry* 140:189–194.

CHAPTER 9

Injury Mortality

C. Mack Sewell
Thomas M. Becker
Charles L. Wiggins
Charles R. Key
Jonathan M. Samet

The high number of deaths from injury in the state of New Mexico is cause for serious concern. New Mexico has the second highest injury mortality rate in the nation—second only to that of Alaska (Baker, O'Neill, and Karpf 1984). The motor vehicle fatality rate in the state, consistently among the nation's highest since 1950, makes a large contribution to the high injury mortality rate (New Mexico Health and Environment Department, Vital Statistics Bureau [VSB] 1984). However, the state is also burdened by high injury mortality rates from many other causes, including both unintentional and intentional injuries. Injuries rank as the third leading cause of death in New Mexico, and as the leading cause of death for persons aged 1 to 44 years (New Mexico Health and Environment Department, VSB 1988).

In 1985, the New Mexico death rate for all injuries was over 60% higher than the U.S. rate (94.4 *versus* 58.1 per 100,000 population) (New Mexico Health and Environment Department, VSB 1986a). Studies to estimate the economic cost of injuries have not been reported for New Mexico; however, national data indicate that between $75 billion and $100 billion are expended each year in the U.S. in direct and indirect costs for injuries (Committee on Trauma Research 1985), suggesting that the costs of injury for New Mexico must be substantial.

To characterize better the total injury problem in New Mexico, we calculated proportionate injury mortality and age-adjusted injury mortality rates by cause for New Mexico's American Indians, Hispanics, and non-Hispanic whites for the years 1958 through 1982. Data are presented for total external mortality and for leading causes of injury mortality, including motor vehicle accidents, suicide, homicide, falls, drowning, and exposure. Suicide and homicide will also be discussed in greater detail in Chapter 10.

Methodologic Considerations

Deaths were assigned to accidents and other external causes if coded as E800–E900.9 in the seventh, eighth, and ninth revisions of the International Classification of Diseases (ICD) (World Health Organization [WHO] 1957, 1967, 1977). Because many cause-specific codes in ICD7, ICD8, and ICD9 were changed, a list of appropriate ICD codes for each revision and for each time period was prepared for classification of deaths and for subsequent analyses (see Appendix).

Results

Total External Mortality

Age-adjusted mortality rates for the total of all external causes varied widely between the sexes and among the three major ethnic groups in New Mexico (Tables 9.1 and 9.2). Males of each ethnic group consistently had higher average annual age-adjusted mortality rates than did females. Among males, American Indians consistently had the highest rates, followed by Hispanics; among females, American Indians had the highest rates, followed by similar rates for Hispanic and non-Hispanic whites. In both sexes, the mortality rates for American Indians were two to three times higher than those for the state's other ethnic groups, and two to five times higher than age-adjusted rates for U.S. whites within comparable time periods.

Leading Causes of Injury Mortality

Of the 10 leading causes of external mortality in New Mexico in the years 1958 through 1982, motor vehicle crashes ranked first for both sexes in all three ethnic groups (Tables 9.3 and 9.4). In the other nine leading causes of external mortality, rates differed substantially among the three ethnic groups, although homicide, suicide, falls, drowning, and fire- and burn-associated deaths all accounted for large numbers of deaths in both sexes in all ethnic groups. Homicide accounted for twice the proportion of deaths in Hispanic than in non-Hispanic white males (12.5% and 6.1%, respectively). Suicide accounted for almost 20% of the deaths from external causes in non-Hispanic white males, nearly twice the 11.5% in Hispanic and 10% in American Indian males. Although airplane crashes accounted for 4.2% of non-Hispanic white male deaths, and were the fifth ranking cause of external mortality in this ethnic

Table 9.1

Mortality rates* in New Mexico males from total external causes, motor vehicle accidents, suicide, and homicide, as compared with selected U.S. rates, 1958 through 1982

Cause of death	Time period (inclusive years)				
	1958–62	1963–67	1968–72	1973–77	1978–82
Total external causes					
Non-Hispanic white	139.3	140.6	143.9	140.8	126.1
Hispanic	145.9	136.9	188.9	179.0	161.2
American Indian	279.6	299.5	438.2	488.9	363.7
U.S. white[a]	95.2	101.1	106.8	97.4	93.2
U.S. black	147.8	166.5	212.6	182.4	162.9
Motor vehicle accidents					
Non-Hispanic white	51.1	50.1	53.0	49.3	49.1
Hispanic	65.8	62.3	78.5	74.7	63.9
American Indian	128.8	122.3	203.4	233.0	166.9
U.S. white	32.3	38.8	39.3	30.9	33.3
U.S. black	36.1	42.2	48.3	34.9	31.8
Suicide					
Non-Hispanic white	23.4	22.9	28.6	28.8	28.6
Hispanic	10.7	10.9	18.2	24.2	25.4
American Indian	25.0	18.7	33.1	48.8	35.7
U.S. white	18.2	18.1	18.3	19.6	18.5
U.S. black	7.4	8.6	9.2	10.6	10.2
Homicide					
Non-Hispanic white	4.1	5.8	6.2	11.1	10.8
Hispanic	11.5	10.4	20.2	23.0	27.5
American Indian	17.2	14.1	29.9	46.5	39.7
U.S. white	3.7	4.4	6.7	8.6	9.9
U.S. black	39.7	48.6	74.0	72.1	63.9

* Age-adjusted rates per 100,000, age-adjusted to the 1970 U.S. population.
[a] Rates for U.S. whites and blacks are calculated for the midpoints of each 5-year interval (1960, 1965, 1970, 1975, 1980).

group, airplane crash-related mortality did not appear in the 10 leading causes of external death for American Indian or Hispanic males. Deaths from excessive cold and exposure or neglect were important causes of mortality among American Indians, but these conditions were not among the 10 leading causes for Hispanics or for non-Hispanic whites. When

Table 9.2

Mortality rates* in New Mexico females from total external causes, motor vehicle accidents, suicide, and homicide, as compared with selected U.S. rates, 1958 through 1982

Cause of death	Time period (inclusive years)				
	1958–62	1963–67	1968–72	1973–77	1978–82
Total external causes					
Non-Hispanic white	50.3	49.4	55.3	56.3	47.8
Hispanic	37.2	39.2	50.8	44.6	38.4
American Indian	70.2	101.5	125.3	119.7	97.8
U.S. white[a]	37.7	40.5	41.2	36.3	33.0
U.S. black[a]	51.7	51.3	48.3	49.9	44.1
Motor vehicle accidents					
Non-Hispanic white	19.1	18.7	20.6	19.0	17.3
Hispanic	14.8	14.4	20.7	19.3	15.5
American Indian	32.1	47.8	67.1	65.5	56.9
U.S. white	10.5	13.9	14.5	11.0	12.1
U.S. black	9.3	12.6	14.6	9.5	8.2
Suicide					
Non-Hispanic white	6.5	6.4	8.2	11.7	8.9
Hispanic	1.8	1.4	3.7	4.0	5.9
American Indian	1.0	1.6	3.1	6.1	2.7
U.S. white	5.1	6.9	6.9	6.9	5.4
U.S. black	1.7	2.3	2.7	2.7	2.1
Homicide					
Non-Hispanic white	1.9	2.0	3.4	5.3	5.1
Hispanic	3.4	2.3	3.3	4.2	4.7
American Indian	5.9	6.7	12.3	12.5	5.3
U.S. white	1.4	1.6	2.1	2.8	3.0
U.S. black	10.3	10.8	13.6	14.8	12.4

* Age-adjusted rates per 100,000, age-adjusted to the 1970 U.S. population.

[a] Rates for U.S. whites and blacks are calculated for the midpoints of each 5-year interval (1960, 1965, 1970, 1975, 1980).

the two categories of excessive cold and of exposure and neglect were combined, the combination comprised the third leading cause of external mortality for American Indian males, and the fourth (with fall-related mortality) for American Indian females.

Studies of injury mortality frequently separate intentional injuries (sui-

Table 9.3

Leading causes of injury mortality for American Indian, Hispanic, and non-Hispanic white males in New Mexico, 1958 through 1982

Rank	Ethnic Group		
	American Indians	Hispanics	Non-Hispanic whites
1	Traffic crashes 1496 (47.4)[a]	Traffic crashes 3200 (42.3)	Traffic crashes 3621 (36.5)
2	Suicide 316 (10.0)	Homicide 946 (12.5)	Suicide 1948 (19.7)
3	Homicide 256 (8.1)	Suicide 875 (11.5)	Falls 627 (6.3)
4	Excessive cold 171 (5.4)	Drowning 348 (4.6)	Homicide 603 (6.1)
5	Drowning 163 (5.2)	Falls 315 (4.2)	Airplane crashes 413 (4.2)
6	Exposure or neglect 112 (3.5)	Poisoning 250 (3.3)	Fires and burns 306 (3.1)
7	Falls 103 (3.3)	Fires and burns 213 (2.8)	Drowning 303 (3.1)
8	Aspiration of food 63 (2.0)	Firearms (accidental) 186 (2.5)	Firearms (accidental) 252 (2.5)
9	Poisoning 58 (1.8)	Aspiration of Food 150 (2.0)	Poisoning 175 (1.8)
10	Fires and burns 21 (0.7)	Struck by falling object 116 (1.5)	Aspiration of food 156 (1.6)
	Other unintentional injury 399 (12.6)	Other unintentional injury 969 (12.8)	Other unintentional injury 1506 (15.2)
Total	3158 (100.0)	7568 (100.0)	9910 (100.0)

Source: Sewell *et al.* 1989, printed with permission.

[a] Percentages of total injury deaths are given in parentheses.

Table 9.4

Leading causes of injury mortality* for American Indian, Hispanic, and non-Hispanic white females in New Mexico, 1958 through 1982

Rank	Ethnic Group		
	American Indians	Hispanics	Non-Hispanic whites
1	Traffic crashes 535 (50.01)	Traffic crashes 819 (41.0)	Traffic crashes 1384 (35.2)
2	Homicide 92 (8.7)	Falls 202 (10.1)	Suicide 667 (17.0)
3	Fires and burns 56 (5.3)	Homicide 193 (9.6)	Falls 656 (16.7)
4	Falls 48 (4.5)	Suicide 178 (8.9)	Homicide 285 (7.2)
5	Suicide 37 (3.5)	Drowning 97 (4.8)	Poisoning 132 (3.4)
6	Excessive cold 29 (2.7)	Fires and burns 96 (4.8)	Fires and burns 128 (3.3)
7	Drowning 28 (2.7)	Aspiration of food 85 (4.3)	Aspiration of food 97 (2.5)
8	Aspiration of food 21 (2.0)	Poisoning 71 (3.6)	Drowning 87 (2.2)
9	Exposure or neglect 19 (1.8)	Firearms (accidental) 28 (1.4)	Airplane crashes 55 (1.4)
10	Poisoning 15 (1.4)	Struck by falling object 5 (0.3)	Firearms (accidental) 32 (0.8)
	Other unintentional injury 176 (16.7)	Other unintentional injury 224 (11.2)	Other unintentional injury 406 (10.3)
Total	1056 (100.0)	1998 (100.0)	3929 (100.0)

Source: Sewell *et al.* 1989, printed with permission.
*Percentages of total injury deaths are given in parentheses.

cide and homicide) from unintentional (or accidental) injuries. In this chapter, we make no distinction between the two categories of injury mortality in our presentation of data in the tables; the discussion does, however, consider the two categories separately.

Intentional Injuries
Suicide: Age-adjusted annual mortality rates for suicide among New Mexico males were highest for American Indians during all but one of the five time periods studied (Table 9.1); the rates for non-Hispanic white males were second, followed by rates for Hispanics. Suicide was the second leading cause of injury mortality (for both intentional and unintentional causes combined) for American Indian and non-Hispanic white males, and the third leading cause for Hispanic males (Table 9.3).

Age-adjusted annual mortality rates for suicide were lower among females than among males (Table 9.2). The rates were highest for non-Hispanic white females, followed by similar rates for Hispanics and American Indians. Suicide was the second leading cause of injury mortality for non-Hispanic white females (Table 9.4), the fourth for Hispanic females, and the fifth for American Indian females. Suicide as an intentional injury-related cause of death is discussed in more detail in the next chapter.

Homicide: American Indians had the highest age-adjusted annual homicide rates among New Mexico males (Table 9.1). The rates were approximately four times higher than rates for U.S. white males within each time period. Hispanic male homicide rates were second highest, followed by non-Hispanic white males. The homicide rates for non-Hispanic white males in New Mexico were comparable to rates for U.S. white males. Homicide was the second leading cause of injury death for Hispanic males, third for American Indian males, and fourth for non-Hispanic white males (Table 9.3).

New Mexico females had lower age-adjusted annual homicide rates than males. Among females, American Indians had the highest rates in each time period, followed by similar rates for Hispanic and non-Hispanic white females. Homicide was the second leading cause of injury mortality for American Indian females, third for Hispanic females, and fourth for non-Hispanic white females. Homicide as an injury-related cause of death is discussed in more detail in the next chapter.

Unintentional Injuries
Motor vehicle accidents: The age-adjusted annual mortality rates for motor vehicle accidents (Tables 9.1 and 9.2) for all ethnic groups in New

Mexico exceeded the rates for U.S. whites. Among males, in the five time periods studied, American Indian rates were from two to more than four times higher than the rates for non-Hispanic whites; the rates for Hispanics were 20% to 50% higher than for non-Hispanic whites. Among females, American Indians had rates that were from two to more than three times higher than the rates for non-Hispanic whites, while the rates for Hispanics were similar to those for non-Hispanic whites.

Motor vehicle crashes accounted for the largest proportion of all injury deaths in New Mexico, and were the leading cause of injury mortality in all of the principal ethnic groups (Tables 9.3 and 9.4). The proportion of injury mortality resulting from motor vehicle crashes varied from a low of approximately 36% in non-Hispanic whites to almost 50% in American Indians.

Falls: Death as the result of falls was also a leading cause of accidental injury death in New Mexico. The mortality rate for accidental falls in New Mexico was lower than the national rate until 1974, when both rates were 7.7 per 100,000, but since that date has exceeded the national rate (New Mexico Health and Environment Department, VSB 1985a).

Among males, mortality as the result of falls was the second leading cause of unintentional injury for non-Hispanic whites, third for Hispanics, and fifth for American Indians (Table 9.3). Among females, mortality from falls was the second leading cause of unintentional injury for Hispanics and non-Hispanic whites, and the third leading cause for American Indians (Table 9.4).

Drowning: In the U.S., drowning was the third overall leading cause of unintentional injury mortality, and the second leading cause for persons up to 44 years of age (National Safety Council 1987). In New Mexico during the 25-year study period, the mortality rates for drowning were consistently higher than the national rates (New Mexico Health and Environment Department, VSB 1986b). Among males, drowning was the second leading cause of unintentional injury death for Hispanics, third for American Indians, and fifth for non-Hispanic whites (Table 9.3). Among females, drowning was the third leading cause of unintentional injury death for Hispanics, fifth for American Indians, and sixth for non-Hispanic whites (Table 9.4).

Excessive cold/exposure or neglect: Mortality resulting from the combined categories of excessive cold and of exposure or neglect was the second leading cause of death from unintentional injury for American Indian males in New Mexico, and was tied with falls as the third leading cause for American Indian females (Tables 9.3 and 9.4). Neither exposure nor excessive cold appeared among the 10 leading causes of injury mortality for Hispanics or non-Hispanic whites.

Discussion

The high rate of injury mortality in New Mexico is a serious public health problem. Injuries are the third ranking cause of death in the state, and the leading cause of years of potential life lost (YPLL) before age 65. Nationally, injury deaths account for over 40% of YPLL before age 65 (Centers for Disease Control 1982); in New Mexico, the proportion is even higher (New Mexico Health and Environment Department, VSB 1985b). Unintentional injuries accounted for the majority of injury mortalities in New Mexico from 1958 through 1982.

Our data show motor vehicle crashes to be the leading cause of injury mortality in New Mexico for all ethnic groups and for both sexes. Several factors contribute to the high motor vehicle fatality rate: high speed (Gallaher *et al.* 1988), low population density (Baker, Whitfield, and O'Neill 1987), low *per capita* income (Baker, Whitfield, and O'Neill 1987), poor road conditions (Wright and Robertson 1976), alcohol impairment of drivers (McCarrol and Haddon 1962), effects of alcohol on accident injuries (Waller *et al.* 1986), and nonuse of seat belts (U.S. Department of Transportation 1984). Although motor vehicle fatality rates have declined in New Mexico during recent years, the rates remain well above the national figures.

Motor vehicle crashes in New Mexico are frequently related to alcohol consumption, with alcohol involved in 55% to 65% of all motor vehicle fatalities. Although data on the proportion of alcohol-involved vehicle fatalities from other states are scant, New Mexico is believed to have one of the highest proportions in the nation (personal communication, New Mexico Traffic Safety Bureau). Disproportionately high use of alcohol among American Indians in New Mexico may contribute to their elevated motor vehicle mortality rates as compared with rates for Hispanics and non-Hispanic whites (New Mexico Health and Environment Department, Office of Epidemiology [OE] 1988).

Intentional injuries (homicide and suicide) accounted for a substantial proportion of externally caused mortality in all ethnic groups in New Mexico. Although the high proportion of suicides in non-Hispanic whites contrasts sharply with that in American Indians and Hispanics, the mortality rates from suicide among American Indian males are substantially greater than those for non-Hispanic whites in the most recent time periods. Furthermore, very high suicide rates have been reported among some young American Indian men, especially young members of the Apache tribe (VanWinkle and May 1986). In the Southwest, homicide rates among young Hispanic men triple the rates for non-Hispanic white men (Centers for Disease Control 1986). A similar pattern is present in New Mexico and will be discussed in the next chapter. The high proportion of deaths in Hispanics as the result of homicides exceeded that of American Indians and non-Hispanic whites, even though actual rates of homicide were highest for American Indians.

Data from the New Mexico Office of the Medical Investigator show that in 1985 approximately one-half of the homicides and suicides in the state were associated with a measurable alcohol level of greater than 0.005% (University of New Mexico 1985). These data also point to the central role of firearms in homicides and suicides in New Mexico.

The many risk factors for fall-related mortality are varied and complex. Both individual health status and environmental factors contribute to accidental falls. Individual health problems (usually associated with advanced age) include impairment of vision, gait, and balance; increased fragility of long bones related to osteoporosis, a loss of bone mass that is greater in females than males and that increases with age; and greater susceptibility to fatal complications following injury (Baker, O'Neill, and Karpf 1984). Contributing environmental factors include icy or wet surfaces, uneven ground, stairs, and loose rugs and clutter (New Mexico Health and Environment Department, VSB 1985a). Certain medicines or drugs have also been associated with falls (Ray *et al.* 1987). New Mexico's accidental fall mortality rate has exceeded the U.S. rate since 1975.

Despite New Mexico's desert environment, the drowning rate is 40% higher than the national rate (Davis, Ledman, and Kilgore 1985). Nationally, drownings in public places primarily occur while the victims are swimming or playing in the water. The second highest figures are for persons falling into the water from shores, docks, or bridges; water transport and recreational boating accidents rank third (National Safety Council 1985). Studies of home drownings indicate that more than one-half occur in swimming pools, about one-fourth in bathtubs, and the remainder in wells, cisterns, cesspools, and other bodies of water (National Safety Council 1985). In New Mexico, more than half of all drowning victims are younger than 25 years, with toddlers and adolescents at greatest risk (Davis, Ledman, and Kilgore 1985). Rates in the state are highest for American Indian males, followed by Hispanic and non-Hispanic white males. From 1980 through 1984, mortality from drowning was over five times higher for males than for females (New Mexico Health and Environment Department, VSB 1986b). Alcohol has consistently been a major contributing risk factor for drowning (Dietz and Baker 1974).

Mortality attributed to exposure and excessive cold in New Mexico occurs almost exclusively among American Indians. In one study (Fleming, Braun, and Sheline 1986), American Indians were found to be 22 times more likely than members of other races to die from exposure. Risk factors for this category include alcohol and geographic location, with the sites of occurrence clustered on short stretches of roads between off-reservation bars and the reservation boundary.

Alcohol abuse is a major public health problem in New Mexico and a strong contributor to injury mortality. According to the National Institute on Alcohol Abuse and Alcoholism (1985), New Mexico ranks second in the nation after Nevada in the rate of alcohol-related mortality. Studies have shown the rate in New Mexico to be twice the national rate for causes of death that are completely attributable to alcohol (i.e. alcoholic psychoses, alcoholic cardiomyopathy, alcoholic polyneuropathy, alcoholic gastritis, and accidental poisoning with alcohol) (New Mexico Health and Environment Department, OE 1986). In New Mexico, alcohol-related mortality rates for American Indians and Hispanics far exceed the rates for non-Hispanic whites. In the 15- to 24-year age group, the rate for American Indians is 50 times greater than for non-Hispanic whites, and the rate for Hispanics is five times greater than for non-Hispanic whites.

Long-term improvements in emergency medical response and care have undoubtedly increased survival from injuries that would have proven fatal only a few years ago. The implementation of regional trauma systems in other states has resulted in significant improvements in trauma care and in reductions of death rates as the result of trauma. New Mexico has only recently implemented a regional trauma care system, and its effect on injury mortality has not yet been evaluated.

Summary

Age-adjusted mortality rates for all external causes vary widely between the sexes and among the major ethnic groups in New Mexico. Over the 25-year study period, males consistently had higher average annual age-adjusted external mortality rates than did females, and American Indians of both sexes had injury mortality rates two to three times higher than rates for the other ethnic groups. Motor vehicle crashes were the leading cause of death from injury for all three ethnic groups. Other important causes of injury mortality were suicide, homicide, drowning, and death from excessive cold or exposure for American Indians; and suicide, homicide, drowning, and falls for Hispanics and non-Hispanic whites. New Mexico's vital statistics data clearly indicate the magnitude of injury-related mortality as a major public health concern in this state.

Appendix

Cause-specific international classification of diseases (ICD) codes for injury-related events, 1958 through 1982

Cause	ICD7 1958–68	ICD8 1969–78	ICD9 1979–82
Total external	E800-962	E800-949	E810-949
Traffic crashes	E810-825	E810-819	E810-819
Homicide	E964, E980-983	E960-969	E960-969
Suicide	E963, E970-979	E950-959	E950-959
Falls	E900-904	E880-887	E880-888
Drowning	E929	E910	E910
Poisoning	E870-888	E850-869	E850-866
Aspiration of food	E921	E911	E911
Fires and burns	E916	E890-899	E890-899
Airplane crashes	E860-866	E840-845	E840-845
Firearms (accidental)	E919	E922	E922
Excessive cold	E932	E901	E901
Exposure or neglect	E933	E904	E904
Struck by falling object	E910	E916	E916

Source: Sewell *et al.* 1989, printed with permission.

REFERENCES

Baker, S. P., B. O'Neill, and R. S. Karpf. 1984. *The injury fact book.* Lexington Books, Lexington, MA: D.C. Heath and Company.

Baker, S. P., R. A. Whitfield, and B. O'Neill. 1987. Geographic variations in mortality from motor vehicle crashes. *N.Engl.J.Med.* 316:1384–1387.

Centers for Disease Control. 1982. Table V. Years of potential life lost, deaths, and death rates, by cause of death, and estimated number of physician contacts, by principal diagnosis, United States. *Morbidity and Mortality Weekly Reports.* 31:599.

———. 1986. *Homicide surveillance: high risk racial and ethnic groups—blacks and Hispanics, 1970 to 1983.* Atlanta, GA: U.S. Department of Health and Human Services.

Committee on Trauma Research, National Research Council and the Institute of Medicine. 1985. *Injury in America.* Washington, DC: National Academy Press.

Davis, S., J. Ledman, and J. Kilgore. 1985. Drownings of children and youth in a desert state. *West.J.Med.* 143:196–201.

Dietz, P. E., and S. P. Baker. 1974. Drowning: epidemiology and prevention. *Am.J.Public Health* 64:303–312.

Fleming, D. W., M. M. Braun, and J. L. Sheline. April 1986. *Prohibition on the reservation: does it contribute to increased Native American injury mortality?* 35th Epidemic Intelligence Service Annual Conference. Centers for Disease Control. Atlanta, GA.

Gallaher, M. M., C. M. Sewell, H. F. Hull, H. Graff, and J. Fenner. April 1988. *Effects of the 65-mph speed limit on interstate fatalities, New Mexico.* Abstract. 37th Epidemic Intelligence Service Annual Conference. Centers for Disease Control. Atlanta, GA.

McCarroll, J. R., and W. Haddon, Jr. 1962. A controlled study of fatal automobile accidents in New York City. *J.Chronic Dis.* 15:811–826.

National Institute on Alcohol Abuse and Alcoholism. September 1985. *County problem indicators, 1975–1980. U.S. alcohol epidemiologic data reference manual.* Vol 3. Washington, DC.

National Safety Council. 1985. *Accident facts.* 1985 ed. Chicago.

———. 1987. *Accident facts.* 1987 ed. Chicago.

New Mexico Health and Environment Department, Office of Epidemiology. March 1986. *Mortality directly related to alcohol in New Mexico, 1980–1984.* Santa Fe, NM.

———. September 1988. *Native American motor vehicle mortality.* Epidemiology report. Santa Fe, NM.

New Mexico Health and Environment Department, Vital Statistics Bureau. January 1984. *Motor vehicle accident fatalities. Monthly vital statistics report.* Santa Fe, NM.

———. April 1, 1985a. *Accidental fall/fracture fatalities. Monthly vital statistics report.* Santa Fe, NM.

———. June 1985b. *New Mexico years of potential life lost. Monthly vital statistics report.* Santa Fe, NM.

———. February 1986a. *Leading causes of death. Monthly vital statistics report.* Santa Fe, NM.

———. May 1986b. *Drownings in New Mexico. Monthly vital statistics report.* Santa Fe, NM.

———. April 1988. *1986 New Mexico selected health statistics.* Santa Fe, NM.

Ray, W. A., M. R. Griffin, W. Schaffner, D. K. Baugh, and J. L. Melton. 1987. Psychotropic drug use and the risk of hip fracture. *N.Engl.J.Med.* 316:363–369.

Sewell, C. M., T. M. Becker, C. L. Wiggins, C. R. Key, H. F. Hull, and J. M. Samet. 1989. Injury mortality in New Mexico's American Indians, Hispanics, and non-Hispanic whites, 1958–1982. *West.J.Med.* 150:708–713.

University of New Mexico School of Medicine, Office of the Medical Investigator. 1985. *Annual report 1985.* Albuquerque, NM.

U.S. Department of Transportation. 1984. National Highway Traffic Safety Administration, final rule, FMVSS 208, occupant crash protection. *Federal Register* 49:28962–29010.

VanWinkle, N. W., and P. A. May. 1986. Native American suicide in New Mexico, 1957–1979: a comparative study. *Human Organization* 45:296–309.

Waller, P. F., J. R. Stewart, A. R. Hansen, J. C. Stutts, C. L. Popkin, and E. A. Rodgman. 1986. The potentiating effects of alcohol on driver injury. *JAMA* 256:1461–1466.

World Health Organization. 1957. *Manual of the International Statistical Classification of Diseases, Injuries, and Causes of Death.* Based on the recommendations of the Seventh Revision Conference, 1955. Geneva, Switzerland: WHO.

———. 1967. *Manual of the International Statistical Classification of Diseases, Injuries, and Causes of Death.* Based on the recommendations of the Eighth Revision Conference, 1965. Geneva, Switzerland: WHO.

———. 1977. *Manual of the International Statistical Classification of Diseases, Injuries, and Causes of Death.* Based on the recommendations of the Ninth Revision Conference, 1975. Geneva, Switzerland: WHO.

Wright, P. H., and L. S. Robertson. 1976. Priorities for roadside hazard notification: a study of 300 fatal roadside object crashes. *Proceedings of the Twentieth Conference of the American Association for Automotive Medicine.* Des Plaines, IL: American Association for Automotive Medicine. 1976:114–117.

CHAPTER 10

Suicide and Homicide

Thomas M. Becker
Charles L. Wiggins
Charles R. Key
Jonathan M. Samet

The epidemiology of violent deaths—both suicides and homicides—has been well described for various populations in the U.S. Many of the research efforts have focused on minority populations, especially blacks. However, published reports of the epidemiology of suicide and homicide in American Indians and in Hispanics in the U.S. have been few. Descriptive reports of suicides among American Indians that have been published in medical, anthropological, and sociological literature have, unfortunately, been limited either by short observation periods, small numbers of cases, or lack of a population-based perspective (Table 10.1).

New Mexico is among the leading states in the nation in both suicide and homicide rates (O'Carroll 1989; Smith, Mercy, and Warren 1985). We have discussed the high proportional mortality from violent deaths in New Mexico's American Indians, Hispanics, and non-Hispanic whites in Chapter 9. In this chapter, we present homicide and suicide data in greater detail, showing time trends and mortality rates for both causes among the state's three principal ethnic groups for the 25-year period 1958 through 1982.

Methodologic Considerations

For suicides, we examined the following codes from the International Classification of Diseases (ICD): E963–963.9 and E970–979.9 in the ICD7 revision (World Health Organization [WHO] 1955); and E950–E959.9 in the ICD8 (WHO 1967) and ICD9 (WHO 1977) revisions. For homicides, we examined codes E964–964.9 and E980–983.9 in the ICD7 revision, and E960–E969.9 in the ICD8 and ICD9 revisions. These

Table 10.1
Published suicide rates for American Indian tribes

Tribe	Rate[a]	Inclusive Years of Study	Reference
Pacific Northwest, combined	28.0	1969	Shore 1972
Navajo	8.3	1954–63	Levy 1965
Navajo	12.8	1968	Miller and Schoenfeld (1971)
Navajo	23.0	1957–79	Van Winkle and May (1986)
Cherokee	11.5	1972–73	Humphrey and Kupferer (1982)
Cherokee	31.1	1974–76	Humphrey and Kupferer (1982)
Lumbee	8.3	1972–73	Humphrey and Kupferer (1982)
Lumbee	10.3	1974–76	Humphrey and Kupferer (1982)
Shoshone	98.0	1961–68	Dizmang et al. (1974)
Cheyenne	48.0	1960–68	Barter and Werst (1970)
Papago	18.0	1967–71	Conrad and Kahn (1974)
Papago	30.0	1969–71	Conrad and Kahn (1974)
U.S. Indian, Eskimo, Aleut	23.1	1967	Ogden, Spector, and Hill (1970)
Arizona-based tribes	16.8	1971–73	Sievers, Cynamon, and Bittker (1975)
Apache	36.0	1974	Everett (1975)
Apache	81.0	1957–79	Van Winkle and May (1986)
Pueblo		1954–62	Levy (1965)
San Felipe	0.0		
Zuñi	2.8		
Acoma	5.0		
Santo Domingo	6.5		
Jemez	8.3		
Taos	16.7		
Laguna	16.9		
Isleta	22.2		
Pueblo, combined	39.5	1957–79	Van Winkle and May (1986)

[a] Rates per 100,000 population.

codes did not include deaths caused by legal intervention or execution. Comparability ratios for suicide were 0.939 between the ICD8 and ICD7 revisions, and 1.00 between the ICD9 and ICD8 revisions (National Center for Health Statistics [NCHS] 1980). Comparability ratios for homicide were 0.993 between the ICD8 and ICD7 revisions, and 1.01 between the ICD8 and ICD9 revisions (NCHS 1968).

Results

Suicides

The data show increasing age-adjusted trends in rates for suicides among both Hispanic males and females and American Indian males and females from 1958 through 1982 (Table 10.2). Rates remained relatively stable among non-Hispanic whites of both sexes over the study period, but were elevated compared with rates for whites nationwide. Suicide rates for males in each major ethnic group were considerably higher than rates for females. American Indian women had the lowest age-adjusted suicide rates of all sex/ethnic groups in the state.

Age-specific rates were extremely high for suicide among American Indian men 15 to 44 years of age (Table 10.3). For young American Indian men between the ages of 15 and 24 years, the rates peaked at 94.8 per 100,000 from 1978 through 1982, showing increases over time for the young American Indian males in this age group. Few suicides were recorded in older age groups (45 years and older) of American Indian men and women. An increase in suicide rates from 1958 through 1982 was also apparent for young Hispanic men between the ages of 15 and 44 years. For non-Hispanic whites, high age-specific suicide rates were

Table 10.2
Suicide rates* in New Mexican Hispanics, American Indians, and non-Hispanic whites, 1958 through 1982

	Time period (inclusive years)				
	1958–62	1963–67	1968–72	1973–77	1978–82
Males					
Non-Hispanic white	23.4	22.9	28.6	28.8	28.6
Hispanic	10.7	10.9	18.2	24.2	25.4
American Indian	25.0	18.7	33.1	48.8	35.7
U.S. white[a]	18.2	18.1	18.3	19.6	18.5
U.S. black[a]	7.4	8.6	9.2	10.6	10.2
Females					
Non-Hispanic white	6.5	6.7	8.2	11.7	8.9
Hispanic	1.8	1.4	3.7	4.0	5.9
American Indian	1.0	1.6	3.1	6.1	2.7
U.S. white[a]	5.1	6.9	6.9	6.9	5.4
U.S. black[a]	1.7	2.3	2.7	2.7	2.1

Source: Adapted from Becker and Samet (1990) with permission.
* Age-adjusted rates per 100,000.
[a] Rates for U.S. whites and blacks are calculated for the midpoints of each 5-year interval (1960, 1965, 1970, 1975, 1980).

Table 10.1
Published suicide rates for American Indian tribes

Tribe	Rate[a]	Inclusive Years of Study	Reference
Pacific Northwest, combined	28.0	1969	Shore 1972
Navajo	8.3	1954–63	Levy 1965
Navajo	12.8	1968	Miller and Schoenfeld (1971)
Navajo	23.0	1957–79	Van Winkle and May (1986)
Cherokee	11.5	1972–73	Humphrey and Kupferer (1982)
Cherokee	31.1	1974–76	Humphrey and Kupferer (1982)
Lumbee	8.3	1972–73	Humphrey and Kupferer (1982)
Lumbee	10.3	1974–76	Humphrey and Kupferer (1982)
Shoshone	98.0	1961–68	Dizmang et al. (1974)
Cheyenne	48.0	1960–68	Barter and Werst (1970)
Papago	18.0	1967–71	Conrad and Kahn (1974)
Papago	30.0	1969–71	Conrad and Kahn (1974)
U.S. Indian, Eskimo, Aleut	23.1	1967	Ogden, Spector, and Hill (1970)
Arizona-based tribes	16.8	1971–73	Sievers, Cynamon, and Bittker (1975)
Apache	36.0	1974	Everett (1975)
Apache	81.0	1957–79	Van Winkle and May (1986)
Pueblo		1954–62	Levy (1965)
San Felipe	0.0		
Zuñi	2.8		
Acoma	5.0		
Santo Domingo	6.5		
Jemez	8.3		
Taos	16.7		
Laguna	16.9		
Isleta	22.2		
Pueblo, combined	39.5	1957–79	Van Winkle and May (1986)

[a] Rates per 100,000 population.

codes did not include deaths caused by legal intervention or execution. Comparability ratios for suicide were 0.939 between the ICD8 and ICD7 revisions, and 1.00 between the ICD9 and ICD8 revisions (National Center for Health Statistics [NCHS] 1980). Comparability ratios for homicide were 0.993 between the ICD8 and ICD7 revisions, and 1.01 between the ICD8 and ICD9 revisions (NCHS 1968).

Results

Suicides

The data show increasing age-adjusted trends in rates for suicides among both Hispanic males and females and American Indian males and females from 1958 through 1982 (Table 10.2). Rates remained relatively stable among non-Hispanic whites of both sexes over the study period, but were elevated compared with rates for whites nationwide. Suicide rates for males in each major ethnic group were considerably higher than rates for females. American Indian women had the lowest age-adjusted suicide rates of all sex/ethnic groups in the state.

Age-specific rates were extremely high for suicide among American Indian men 15 to 44 years of age (Table 10.3). For young American Indian men between the ages of 15 and 24 years, the rates peaked at 94.8 per 100,000 from 1978 through 1982, showing increases over time for the young American Indian males in this age group. Few suicides were recorded in older age groups (45 years and older) of American Indian men and women. An increase in suicide rates from 1958 through 1982 was also apparent for young Hispanic men between the ages of 15 and 44 years. For non-Hispanic whites, high age-specific suicide rates were

Table 10.2

Suicide rates* in New Mexican Hispanics, American Indians, and non-Hispanic whites, 1958 through 1982

	Time period (inclusive years)				
	1958–62	1963–67	1968–72	1973–77	1978–82
Males					
Non-Hispanic white	23.4	22.9	28.6	28.8	28.6
Hispanic	10.7	10.9	18.2	24.2	25.4
American Indian	25.0	18.7	33.1	48.8	35.7
U.S. white[a]	18.2	18.1	18.3	19.6	18.5
U.S. black[a]	7.4	8.6	9.2	10.6	10.2
Females					
Non-Hispanic white	6.5	6.7	8.2	11.7	8.9
Hispanic	1.8	1.4	3.7	4.0	5.9
American Indian	1.0	1.6	3.1	6.1	2.7
U.S. white[a]	5.1	6.9	6.9	6.9	5.4
U.S. black[a]	1.7	2.3	2.7	2.7	2.1

Source: Adapted from Becker and Samet (1990) with permission.
* Age-adjusted rates per 100,000.
[a] Rates for U.S. whites and blacks are calculated for the midpoints of each 5-year interval (1960, 1965, 1970, 1975, 1980).

Table 10.3
Age-specific suicide rates* in New Mexican non-Hispanic white, Hispanic, and American Indian males, 1958 through 1982

	Time period (inclusive years)				
	1958–62	1963–67	1968–72	1973–77	1978–82
Non-Hispanic white					
15–24 years	16.3	13.5	26.3	38.4	32.4
25–34 years	20.5	21.3	24.1	30.6	36.4
35–44 years	33.2	35.3	29.5	28.3	32.2
Hispanic					
15–24 years	9.0	16.4	31.2	33.7	45.9
25–34 years	17.7	17.3	21.9	39.3	49.6
35–44 years	7.6	20.0	24.3	46.5	37.2
American Indian					
15–24 years	20.8	33.1	66.7	92.4	94.8
25–34 years	70.6	28.0	77.1	79.5	61.2
35–44 years	36.8	42.9	36.4	79.4	61.7

Source: Adapted from Becker and Samet (1990) with permission.
* Rates per 100,000 for selected age groups.

observed among older men (aged 45 years and above), with the highest age-specific rates (75.7 per 100,000) recorded for elderly men from 1978 through 1982 (data not shown). Although non-Hispanic white males aged 15 to 34 years showed increasing suicide rates over the 25-year period of our study, the increase was not as dramatic as for Hispanic and American Indian males. For non-Hispanic white females, suicide rates were consistently higher than rates for Hispanic and American Indian females, with the highest rates among women aged 40 to 55 years (data not shown).

Homicides

Homicide rates increased from 1958 through 1982 for males in all New Mexico ethnic groups (Table 10.4). American Indian and Hispanic men showed elevated homicide rates compared with the state's non-Hispanic whites and with whites nationwide. American Indian women had the highest homicide rates for women of all three ethnic groups within each time period. Age-adjusted homicide rates for all ethnic populations in New Mexico were, however, lower than for U.S. blacks.

Age-specific data showed that American Indian men aged 15 to 54 years were at high homicide risk, with maximum rates of 130 per 100,000 for

Table 10.4
Homicide rates* in New Mexican Hispanics, American Indians, and non-Hispanic whites, 1958 through 1982

	Time period (inclusive years)				
	1958–62	1963–67	1968–72	1973–77	1978–82
Males					
Non-Hispanic white	4.1	5.8	6.2	11.1	10.8
Hispanic	11.5	10.4	20.2	23.0	27.5
American Indian	17.2	14.1	29.9	46.5	39.7
U.S. white[a]	3.7	4.4	6.7	8.6	9.9
U.S. black[a]	39.7	48.6	74.0	72.1	63.9
Females					
Non-Hispanic white	1.9	2.0	3.4	5.3	5.1
Hispanic	3.4	2.3	3.3	4.2	4.7
American Indian	5.9	6.7	12.3	12.5	5.3
U.S. white[a]	1.4	1.6	2.1	2.8	3.0
U.S. black[a]	10.3	10.8	13.6	14.8	12.4

Source: Adapted from Becker and Samet (1990) with permission.
* Age-adjusted rates per 100,000.
[a] Rates for U.S. whites and blacks are calculated for the midpoints of each 5-year interval (1960, 1965, 1970, 1975, 1980).

men aged 45 to 54 years from 1973 through 1977 (Table 10.5). Increasing age-specific homicide rates were observed among American Indian men aged 15 to 54 years over the study period. Age-specific rates were substantially lower for American Indian women than for American Indian men (data not shown). For Hispanic men, age-specific homicide rates were high for males aged 15 to 44 years, and rates increased consistently for most age groups from 1958 through 1982. In contrast, our study showed that homicide rates among Hispanic women were low for all age groups. For non-Hispanic white males, homicide rates were much lower than for American Indian and Hispanic males within most age groups throughout the span of the study. Age-specific homicide rates for non-Hispanic white women were also low, and were comparable with the rates for Hispanic women.

Discussion

Suicides
Our data clearly indicate that suicide is a substantial problem in New Mexico, and a major source of years of potential life lost, especially

Table 10.5
Age-specific homicide rates* in New Mexican Hispanic, American Indian, and non-Hispanic white males, 1958 through 1982

	Time period (inclusive years)				
	1958–62	1963–67	1968–72	1973–77	1978–82
Non-Hispanic white					
15–24 years	2.8	4.2	5.7	14.6	16.9
25–34 years	5.1	6.1	8.7	21.4	15.9
35–44 years	9.7	12.6	12.3	19.1	18.7
45–54 years	7.0	8.9	8.6	14.2	10.9
Hispanic					
15–24 years	21.2	16.9	32.7	35.5	38.2
25–34 years	15.9	18.0	35.3	48.1	64.8
35–44 years	16.3	16.9	24.3	44.7	56.6
45–54 years	15.6	16.2	26.0	17.5	24.6
American Indian					
15–24 years	27.7	10.2	53.9	37.4	51.7
25–34 years	10.9	24.0	32.5	58.7	74.5
35–44 years	14.7	24.5	48.5	58.3	57.3
45–54 years	20.2	26.6	60.6	130.0	66.1

Source: Adapted from Becker and Samet (1990) with permission.
* Rates per 100,000 for selected age groups.

among younger American Indian men. Suicide is the second leading cause of injury mortality in American Indian men in the state, with 90% of suicides among American Indians from 1958 through 1982 occurring among males (see Chapter 8). This sex ratio among American Indians varies substantially from the non-Hispanic white suicide ratio, which is approximately three males to one female. However, reports from American Indian tribes in other states have shown suicide rates to be equal in both sexes (Andre and Ghachu 1975; Conrad and Kahn 1974; Dizmang et al. 1974; Levy 1965; Webb and Willard 1975). Reports on the Zuñi in New Mexico and on Northwest Coast tribes in the U.S. have shown that men in these tribes attempt and complete suicide at higher rates than do women (Andre and Ghachu 1975; Shore et al. 1972); however, in a study of the White Mountain Apache of Arizona, Levy and Kunitz (1969) reported that more women than men in that tribe committed suicide.

As we discussed in earlier chapters, the social, cultural, and economic characteristics of New Mexico's American Indian population vary substantially from those of the state's Hispanic and non-Hispanic white populations (U.S. Bureau of the Census 1982; Ortiz 1983). A large proportion of the state's American Indians live below the poverty level (U.S. Bureau of the Census 1982). Our vital statistics data cannot address the potential effects of cultural and economic factors as they may affect high suicide rates; however, many of these issues have been discussed by other researchers (Berlin 1987; Havinghurst 1971; Levy 1965; VanWinkle and May 1986).

Consistently recorded information on the methods of suicide among American Indians is not available. However, Sheline and coworkers (1986) showed that an increasing proportion of New Mexico's American Indian men have committed suicide by hanging. Their study also showed that incarceration in jails, especially in nonreservation jails, was a strong risk factor for committing suicide.

Among the Hispanic population in New Mexico, suicide is the third leading cause of injury-related mortality (see Chapter 9). Our data suggest that this cause of death among Hispanics is becoming reason for ever greater concern. An increasing rate of suicides was observed from 1958 through 1982, with rates for Hispanic males far surpassing those for Hispanic females (approximately 5:1 for each 5-year period). As with American Indian women, Hispanic women in New Mexico were at low suicide risk compared with non-Hispanic white women (Table 10.2). Traditional social support systems with family dynamics focused around an older female may be an influence in the lower suicide rates in both Hispanic and American Indian women, especially older women (Gonzales 1967; Ortiz 1983). Age-specific patterns of suicides in Hispanics were comparable to patterns seen in American Indians, although for most age and sex groups, rates were lower in Hispanics than in American Indians. Like young American Indian men, young Hispanic men between the ages of 15 and 34 years were at increased risk for suicide.

Among non-Hispanic whites in New Mexico, suicide was the second leading cause of injury-related death from 1958 through 1982 (see Chapter 9). Age-adjusted suicide rates among non-Hispanic whites of both sexes exceeded Hispanic rates throughout the study period. Rates for non-Hispanic white women also exceeded rates for American Indian and Hispanic women for each 5-year period of this study. Our data show dramatic differences between the age-specific suicide rates among the state's non-Hispanic whites—especially males—and those among minority populations of the state. Although a broader age range of younger non-Hispanic white males was at high risk for suicide (Table 10.3), the highest age-specific rates were observed among men aged 70 years and above (data not shown). These observations are consistent with national data, which indicate that older white men are at increased suicide risk (Monk 1987). For non-Hispanic white women, our age-specific statistics are also comparable to patterns for white women nationwide, with elevated rates observed for middle-aged women between 40 and 55 years (Monk 1987; NCHS 1967).

Homicides

Homicide is a leading cause of injury-related death among American Indians in New Mexico (see Chapter 9). However, the high rate of homicides among American Indians is not peculiar to the State of New Mexico. National data for 1980 indicate that the homicide rates for American Indians, Aleuts, and Eskimos were among the highest in the country, with rates for American Indians 70% higher than those for whites (CDC 1987b). Although American Indians constituted 12% of the nation's nonblack minority population in 1982 (U.S. Bureau of the Census 1982), homicides among American Indians accounted for 43% of all homicides in the nonblack minority group (CDC 1987b). In several northern states with large American Indian populations—Alaska, Montana, North Dakota, and South Dakota—homicide rates among various tribes were significantly elevated compared with rates among whites (CDC 1987b). In the Tucson Indian Health Service Area, homicide accounted for 10% of all injury-related mortality in 1985, while among the Sioux in South Dakota, homicide was the second leading cause of injury-related death (Smith *et al.* in press). Indian Health Service data collected from 1980 through 1982 also indicate elevated rates of homicide among numerous tribes compared with national rates for all races (Office of Technology Assessment [OTA] 1986). New Mexico's statistics parallel the national data for American Indians and, furthermore, show an increase in rates among males over the 25-year span of our study.

Homicide was the second leading injury-related cause of death among Hispanics in New Mexico from 1958 through 1982 (see Chapter 9). A published summary of data from the National Center for Health Statistics for 1970 through 1983 indicates that rates of homicide among Hispanics in the Southwest are three times as high as for non-Hispanic whites (CDC 1987a). Our data for New Mexico are consistent with that report, and also show that the increased risk for Hispanics was mainly among males. The age groups at highest risk among Hispanics included men between the ages of 15 and 55 years. Although New Mexico statistics do not indicate the method of homicide among Hispanics, reports from the New Mexico Office of the Medical Investigator (OMI) (New Mexico OMI 1986) indicate that firearms were associated with homicides among

Hispanics in more than half the cases. National data show that Hispanic homicide victims were killed by firearms in approximately 65% of the cases (CDC 1987a).

Published data that specifically address homicides among non-Hispanic whites in the U.S. are few. Most homicide reports have focused on minority groups, and have included Hispanics and non-Hispanic whites under the single category "white." Whites in New Mexico (Hispanic and non-Hispanic combined) were shown to have the nation's highest homicide rate among whites in 1980—18 per 100,000 (O'Carroll and Mercy 1989). Our data suggest that this rate elevation is due mainly to the high Hispanic rates, which were approximately two- to threefold higher than non-Hispanic white rates among both men and women throughout most of our study period (Table 10.4). New Mexico's homicide rates for non-Hispanic whites were generally comparable to national rates for whites throughout the study period, 1958 through 1982; however, the rates for women in the state almost doubled the national rates for women from 1973 through 1982. As in the rest of the nation, firearms were the weapon most commonly used in homicides in New Mexico (New Mexico OMI 1986).

We discussed in earlier chapters the potential sources of bias in studies of ethnic differences in cause-specific death rates. Additional sources of bias must also be considered in studies of both suicide and homicide. Suicides are particularly subject to inaccurate determination, and the incidence of suicide may be underestimated by 10% to 50% (Jobes, Berman, and Josselson 1987; Litman 1980; NCHS 1967; Toolan 1975). The underestimation of suicide rates may result from lack of criteria for a coroner's determination of suicide as the cause of death, or from lack of specific operational definitions of suicide (O'Carroll 1988; Rosenberg *et al.* 1988). Inability to recognize certain motor vehicle and other injury-related causes of death as suicide also complicates interpretation of the data (Schmidt *et al.* 1977). For both suicides and homicides, under-reporting of deaths is problematic from the perspective of legal jurisdiction to investigate cases. In New Mexico, the OMI examines all cases of suicide and homicide on nonreservation or nonfederal lands, but must be legally invited to participate in the medical/legal investigation of cases on American Indian reservations. Violent deaths on reservation lands are, therefore, more likely to be underreported than are cases outside reservation lands. In addition, homicides or suicides before 1974 were less likely to be thoroughly investigated than were cases reported after the establishment of the OMI in 1974. In a rural state such as New Mexico, many bodies of suicide and homicide victims are not immediately recovered, and may be among the many corpses that are discovered in remote areas of the state without clear signs of cause of death (New Mexico OMI 1986).

Despite these potential sources of bias in the New Mexico vital data on suicide and homicide, our analyses demonstrate the magnitude of the problem of violent deaths in New Mexico. As with blacks nationwide (CDC 1987a, 1988, 1989; Gulaid *et al.* 1988), Hispanics in other southwestern states (CDC 1987a; Smith, Mercy, and Warren 1985), and American Indians in tribes outside New Mexico (CDC 1987b; OTA 1986, U.S. Department of Health and Human Services 1985;), the minority populations of New Mexico are at high risk for violent death. Observed trends in both suicide and homicide data for minority males in New Mexico indicate that their rates of violent death will increase through the next decades unless effective preventive strategies can be put into place.

Summary

Our data revealed high age-adjusted rates for both suicides and homicides among Hispanic and American Indian males in comparison with rates for non-Hispanic white males. Suicide rates among American Indian women were comparatively low, contrasting with their high homicide rates. Homicide rates for males in all three New Mexico ethnic groups increased substantially over the 25-year study period. We conclude that death from violent causes, both suicide and homicide, is a major public health problem in New Mexico, and disproportionately affects minority males.

REFERENCES

Andre, J. M., and S. Ghachu. 1975. *Suicidal occurrence in an American Indian community.* Unpublished manuscript. U.S. Public Health Service, Albuquerque Area Office, Division of Indian Health.

Barter, J. T., and K. M. Werst. 1970. *Historical and contemporary patterns of Northern Cheyenne suicide.* Annual meeting of the American Psychiatric Association, San Francisco, 1970.

Becker, T. M., and J. M. Samet, C. L. Wiggins, and C. R. Key. 1990. Violent death in the West: suicide and homicide in New Mexico, 1958–1987. *Suicide Life Threat.Behav.* 20:324–334.

Berlin, J. D. 1987. Suicide among American Indian adolescents: an overview. *Suicide Life Threat.Behav.* 17:218–232.

Centers for Disease Control. 1987a. Homicide surveillance: high risk racial and ethnic groups—blacks and Hispanics, 1970–1983. *Morbidity and Mortality Weekly Reports* 36:634–640.

———. 1987b. Injuries in an Indian community—Cherokee, North Carolina. *Morbidity and Mortality Weekly Reports* 36:779–781.
———. 1988. Operational criteria for determining suicide. *Morbidity and Mortality Weekly Reports* 37:773–779.
———. 1989. Impact of homicide on YPLL in Michigan's black population. *Morbidity and Mortality Weekly Reports* 38:4–10.
Conrad, R. D., and M. W. Kahn. 1974. An epidemiological study of suicide and attempted suicide among the Papago Indians. *Am.J.Psychiatry* 131:69–72.
Dizmang, L H., J. Watson, P. A. May, and J. Bopp. 1974. Adolescent suicide at an Indian reservation. *Am.J.Orthopsychiatry* 44:43–49.
Everett, M. W. 1975. American Indian social pathology—a re-examination. *Psychological Anthropology* 1975:249–285.
Gonzales, N. L. 1967. *The Spanish Americans of New Mexico.* Albuquerque, NM: University of New Mexico Press.
Gulaid, J. A., E. C. O. Saunders, J. J. Sacks, and D. R. Roberts. 1988. Differences in death rates due to injury among blacks and whites, 1984. *Morbidity and Mortality Weekly Reports* 37:25–32.
Havinghurst, R. J. 1971. The extent and significance of suicide among American Indians today. *Mental Hygiene* 55:174–177.
Humphrey, J. A., and H. J. Kupferer. 1982. Homicide and suicide among the Cherokee and Lumbee Indians of North Carolina. *Int.J.Social Psychiatry* 28:121–128.
Jobes, D. A., A. L. Berman, and A. R. Josselson. 1987. Improving the validity and reliability of medical-legal certifications of suicide. *Suicide Life Threat. Behav.* 17:310–325.
Levy, J. E. 1967. Navajo suicide. *Human Organization* 24:308–318.
Levy, J. E., and S. J. Kunitz. 1969. Notes on some White Mountain Apache social pathologies. *Plateau* 42:11–19.
Litman, R. 1980. Psycho-legal aspects of suicide. In *Modern legal medicine: psychiatry and forensic sciences,* edited by W. Curran, A. L. McGarry, and C. S. Petty, 841–853. Philadelphia: F. A. Davis Co.
Miller, S. I., and L. S. Schoenfeld. 1971. Suicide attempt patterns among the Navajo Indians. *Int.J.Social Psychiatry* 17:189–193.
Monk, M. 1987. Epidemiology of suicide. *Epidemiologic Reviews* 9:51–69.
National Center for Health Statistics. 1967. *Suicide in the United States, 1950–1964.* PHS Publication No. 1000, Series 20, No. 5. Washington, DC: U.S. Department of Health, Education, and Welfare, Public Health Service.
———. 1968. *Provisional estimates of the selected comparability ratio based on dual coding of 1966 death certificates by the seventh and eighth revisions of the International Classification of Diseases.* Washington, DC: U.S. Government Printing Office.
———. 1980. *Estimates of the comparability ratio based on dual coding of 1976 death certificates by the eighth and ninth revisions of the International Classification of Diseases.* Washington, DC: U.S. Government Printing Office.
New Mexico Office of the Medical Investigator. 1986. *Office of the Medical In-*

vestigator Yearly Report, 1986. Albuquerque, NM: New Mexico State Laboratory Division.

O'Carroll, P. W. 1988. Homicides among black males 15–24 years of age, 1970–1984. *Morbidity and Mortality Weekly Reports* 37:53–60.

O'Carroll, P. W., and J. A. Mercy. 1989. Regional variation on homicide rates: why is the West so violent? *Violence and Victims* 4:17–25.

Office of Technology Assessment. 1986. *Indian health care.* Department of Health and Human Services. Washington, DC: U.S. Government Printing Office.

Ogden, M., M. I. Spector, and C. A. Hill. 1970. Suicide and homicides among Indians. *Public Health Report* 85:75–80.

Ortiz, A., ed. 1983. *Handbook of North American Indians.* Vol. 9, *Southwest.* Smithsonian Institution. Washington, DC: U.S. Government Printing Office.

Rosenberg, M. L., L. E. Davidson, J. C. Smith, A. L. Berman, H. Busbee, G. Gantner, G. A. Gay, B. Moore-Lewis, D. H. Mills, D. Murray, P. W. O'Carroll, and D. Jobes. 1988. Operational criteria for the determination of suicide. *J.Forensic Sci.* 33:1445–1456.

Schmidt, C. W., J. W. Shaffer, H. I. Zlotowitz, and R. S. Fisher. 1977. Suicide by vehicular crash. *Am.J.Psychiatry.* 134:175–178.

Sheline, J., T. M. Becker, A. Ortiz, and H. F. Hull. April 1986. *Suicide by hanging: an epidemic among Native Americans?* Abstract. Epidemic Intelligence Service meeting. Atlanta, GA.

Shore, J. H., 1972. Suicide and suicide attempts among American Indians of the Pacific Northwest. *Int.J.Social Psychiatry* 18:91–96.

Shore, J. H., J. F. Bopp, T. R. Waller, and J. W. Dawes. 1972. A suicide prevention center on an Indian Reservation. *Am.J.Psychiatry* 128:76–81.

Sievers, M. L., M. H. Cynamon, and T. E. Bittker. 1975. Intentional isoniazid overdosage among Southwestern American Indians. *Am.J.Psychiatry* 136:662–665.

Smith, J. C., J. A. Mercy, and C. W. Warren. 1985. Comparison of suicides among Anglos and Hispanics in five Southwestern states. *Suicide Life Threat.Behav.* 15:14–26.

Smith, S. M., B. K. Molloy, H. J. Winick, and P. L. Graitcer. 1992. Rural American Indian injury patterns. *J.Environ.Health.* 54:22–25.

Toolan, J. M. 1975. Suicide in children and adolescents. *Am.J.Psychotherapy.* 29:339–344.

U.S. Bureau of the Census. 1982. *Census of the population, 1980.* Washington, DC: U.S. Government Printing Office.

U.S. Department of Health and Human Services. 1985. *Report of the Secretary's Task Force on Black and Minority Health.* Washington, DC: U.S. Department of Health and Human Services, Public Health Service.

VanWinkle, N., and P. May. 1986. Native American suicide in New Mexico: a comparative study. *Human Organization* 45:296–309.

Webb, J. P., and W. Willard. 1975. Six American Indian patterns of suicide. In

Suicide in different cultures, edited by N. L. Farberow, 17–33. Baltimore, MD: University Park Press.

World Health Organization. 1957. *Manual of the International Statistical Classification of Diseases, Injuries, and Causes of Death.* Based on the recommendations of the Seventh Revision Conference, 1955. Geneva, Switzerland: WHO.

———. 1967. *Manual of the International Statistical Classification of Diseases, Injuries, and Causes of Death.* Based on the recommendations of the Eighth Revision Conference, 1965. Geneva, Switzerland: WHO.

———. 1977. *Manual of the International Statistical Classification of Diseases, Injuries, and Causes of Death.* Based on the recommendations of the Ninth Revision Conference, 1975. Geneva, Switzerland: WHO

CHAPTER 11

Symptoms, Signs, and Ill-Defined Conditions:
A Leading Cause of Death Among Minorities

Thomas M. Becker
Charles Wiggins
Charles R. Key
Jonathan M. Samet

The International Classification of Diseases includes the category "symptoms, signs, and ill-defined conditions" for deaths not attributable to a more specific category. We questioned whether a death is more likely to be assigned to this category for persons with no known medical history, or who have not regularly or recently received care from a physician or clinic. People in this group tend to be economically disadvantaged or to live in medically underserved areas; they may also include those who elect to use alternate healing methods. These people are less likely to receive consistent medical care than are those who can afford to use, and elect to use, the conventional medical care system (U.S. Department of Health and Human Services 1982; U.S. Bureau of the Census 1981). When an individual dies in isolation from the medical community, the cause of death may be difficult to establish, particularly if an autopsy is not performed. We hypothesized that, without physician knowledge of the decedent's previous health status, and in absence of an autopsy, the death certificate is more likely to be coded with a "cause unknown" code such as "natural causes" or "death with no signs of disease," which the state nosologist will eventually assign to the category "symptoms, signs, and ill-defined conditions."

We further speculated that "symptoms, signs, and ill-defined conditions" may be given more frequently as the category of death among

Table 11.1
Crude death rates* from symptoms, signs, and ill-defined conditions for leading states, 1980

State	Overall	White	Black
Mississippi	57.2	34.4	99.2
Alabama	53.8	48.5	100.7
Arkansas	39.2	32.8	80.0
Missouri	38.7	38.5	44.3
New Mexico	34.8	40.2	—[a]
Pennsylvania	22.8	15.2	103.0
Texas	22.3	23.3	32.5
South Carolina	19.4	13.7	32.9
Tennessee	17.9	16.5	26.0
Idaho	17.5	18.2	—[a]
U.S. average	12.7	—	—

Source: Becker *et al.* (1989b), printed with permission.
* Rates per 100,000.
[a] Fewer than 10 cases reported.

minority populations in New Mexico than among the non-Hispanic white majority. National vital statistics data indicate that blacks have higher mortality rates attributed to this category than do whites (World Health Organization 1957), and also show that states which include large proportions of blacks in their censuses have higher rates of mortality attributed to this category (Table 11.1). However, the rates and patterns of mortality ascribed to "symptoms, signs, and ill-defined conditions" (referred to hereafter without the quotation marks) have not been described for minority groups other than blacks in the U.S. Accordingly, we examined ethnic differences in mortality attributed to this category in New Mexico. Our findings are presented in this chapter.

Methodologic Considerations

Symptoms, signs, and ill-defined conditions included Codes 780 to 799 in all three revisions of the International Classification of Diseases (ICD), spanning the period 1958 through 1982.

In addition to calculating age-adjusted and age-specific rates for the entire state, we also examined differences in rates of mortality attributed to this category in urban and rural counties in New Mexico. For this calculation, we determined age-adjusted mortality rates for the three New Mexico counties with urban population centers of 50,000 or greater in 1980 and for the other (rural) counties.

We have used ischemic heart disease mortality as an example to demonstrate the potential bias in mortality rate calculations that can result from assignment of deaths to symptoms, signs, and ill-defined conditions. For these calculations, we examined deaths attributed to ischemic heart disease from 1978 through 1982. The ICD codes included ICD 410–413 in the eighth revision for 1978, and ICD 410–414.9 in the ninth revision for 1979 through 1982. To control for artifactual decreases in ischemic heart disease mortality associated with ICD coding changes, we adjusted the numbers of cases of ischemic heart disease-related deaths as described in Chapter 6 (Becker *et al.* 1988). We then calculated age-adjusted and age-specific (for age group 75 years old and above) mortality rates from ischemic heart disease for the period 1978 through 1982. In the next step, we combined the numbers of deaths attributed to ischemic heart disease with those attributed to symptoms, signs, and ill-defined conditions coded over the same time span, 1978 through 1982. We recalculated the age-adjusted and age-specific rates, recording the changes in ischemic heart disease mortality rates that resulted from the addition of cases ascribed to symptoms, signs, and ill-defined conditions.

Results

Age-adjusted mortality rates for deaths attributed to symptoms, signs, and ill-defined conditions among all three principal ethnic groups in New Mexico exceeded the national rates for whites. Differences were most pronounced for American Indians, for whom the mortality rates in both sexes exceeded the rates for Hispanics and non-Hispanic whites in each study period. The mortality rate from this same category for American Indian women was 21-fold higher than the national rate for white women in the period 1963 through 1967 (Table 11.2). Mortality rates from symptoms, signs, and ill-defined conditions for New Mexico's Hispanic men from 1958 through 1962 were tenfold higher than national rates for white men. Mortality rates for Hispanics consistently exceeded rates for non-Hispanic whites in the state.

Time trends of decreasing mortality attributed to symptoms, signs, and ill-defined conditions were apparent for each sex and ethnic group in New Mexico across the entire period 1958 through 1982, except for non-Hispanic white women. For the non-Hispanic white women, mortality rates increased by almost half over the 25-year study period. On the national level, mortality rates attributed to this category over the en-

Table 11.2
Mortality rates* in New Mexicans attributed to symptoms, signs, and ill-defined conditions, by ethnic group and sex, 1958 through 1982

	Time period (inclusive years)				
	1958–62	1963–67	1968–72	1973–77	1978–82
Males					
Non-Hispanic white	58.3	42.9	31.9	49.1	49.2
Hispanic	95.3	80.8	52.3	56.9	58.3
American Indian	155.1	173.3	129.5	139.4	115.6
U.S. white	11.0	12.0	12.9	15.7	13.1
U.S. black	49.1	49.6	53.2	54.0	41.3
Females					
Non-Hispanic white	18.9	16.8	17.7	23.9	27.9
Hispanic	64.9	40.9	27.9	31.1	30.9
American Indian	105.0	138.1	93.4	80.4	81.7
U.S. white	6.3	6.4	6.8	8.6	7.6
U.S. black	36.3	34.7	34.8	32.5	25.0

Source: Becker *et al.* (1989b), printed with permission.
* Age-adjusted rates per 100,000.

tire study period increased among whites but decreased among blacks.

We also calculated age-specific mortality rates attributed to symptoms, signs, and ill-defined conditions for each ethnic and gender group. For each group, rates were highest for persons aged 75 years and older (Figures 11.1 through 11.6). For most cohorts, age-specific mortality declined from the earliest period and rose at the end of the period. Age-specific mortality rates by birth cohort were highest in American Indians, followed by Hispanics and non-Hispanic whites. Rates were consistently higher in males than in females in each ethnic group.

An analysis of mortality rates attributed to symptoms, signs, and ill-defined conditions for differences between urban and rural counties in New Mexico showed the age-adjusted rates in the three urban counties to be comparable to rates observed in all the rural counties combined. We did not find differences within sex or ethnic groups when the age-adjusted rates were compared by urban and rural status.

To describe the extent of bias that can be caused by classification of deaths as due to symptoms, signs, and ill-defined conditions, we adjusted mortality from ischemic heart disease by combining deaths attributed to symptoms, signs, and ill-defined conditions with those attributed to

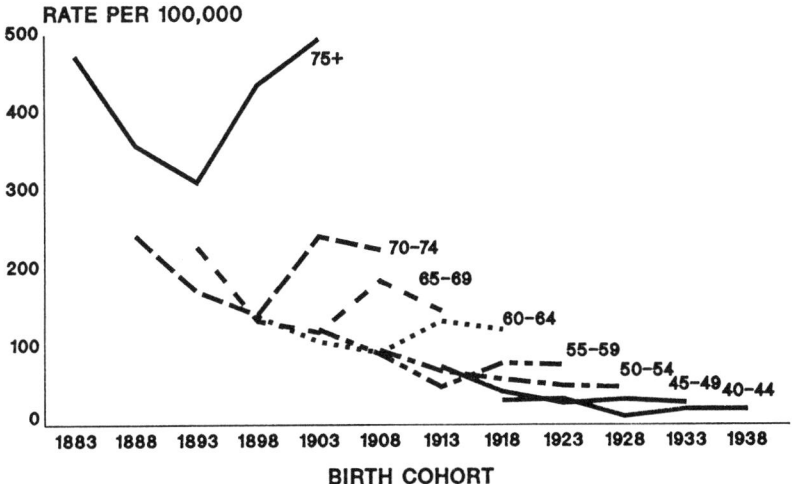

Figure 11.1. *Mortality from symptoms, signs, and ill-defined conditions among non-Hispanic white males in New Mexico, by 5-year birth cohort.*

ischemic heart disease in New Mexico from 1978 through 1982. Age-adjusted mortality rates from ischemic heart disease among American Indians, Hispanics, and non-Hispanic whites increased as a result of the combined cause-of-death calculations (Table 11.3). The amount of increase varied with the proportion of deaths ascribed to symptoms, signs, and ill-defined conditions added to ischemic heart disease deaths. The magnitude of increase in age-adjusted rates was greater for American Indians than for Hispanics and non-Hispanic whites.

The potential bias from assignment of deaths to symptoms, signs, and ill-defined conditions was further examined for persons 75 years and older—the age group with the highest mortality rate from this nonspecific grouping. Substantial changes in age-specific rates of ischemic heart disease among elderly New Mexicans were also observed as a result of combining deaths from ischemic heart disease and those assigned to symptoms, signs, and ill-defined conditions (Table 11.4). As with age-adjusted mortality rates, age-specific mortality rates for ischemic heart disease shifted most dramatically for American Indians.

SYMPTOMS, SIGNS MORTALITY
NON–HISPANIC WHITE FEMALES

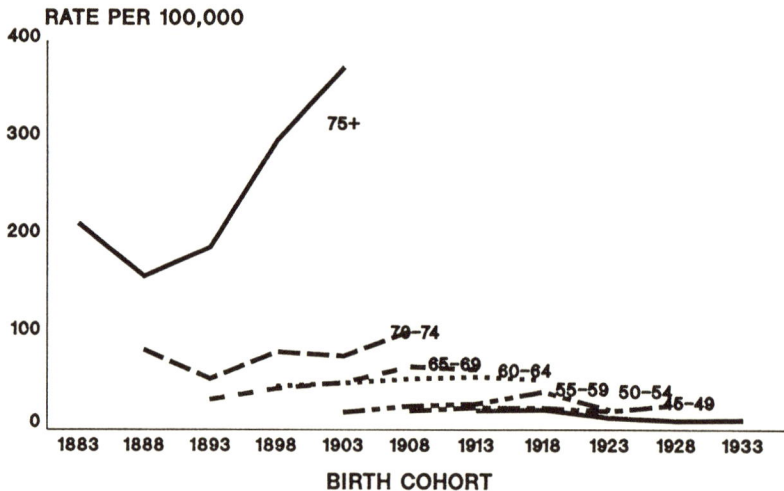

Figure 11.2. *Mortality from symptoms, signs, and ill-defined conditions among non-Hispanic white females in New Mexico, by 5-year birth cohort.*

Discussion

In New Mexico, the risk of death attributed to symptoms, signs, and ill-defined conditions far exceeded the risk for all U.S. whites. Mortality rates from this category among American Indians were enormous compared with the rates in New Mexico whites and in whites nationwide. The rate for Hispanics was also very high compared to the rate for whites nationwide.

Mortality rates for many diseases among New Mexico's non-Hispanic whites are comparable to national rates for whites (Becker *et al.* 1988, 1989a; Wiggins *et al.* 1989; Samet *et al.* 1980, 1988; Key 1981); in contrast, mortality rates attributed to symptoms, signs, and ill-defined conditions in the state's non-Hispanic whites nearly tripled the national rates for whites (Becker *et al.* 1989b). Moreover, for the minority populations in New Mexico, the attribution of deaths to this category was a leading "cause" of mortality, and for American Indians, it far exceeded mortality from ischemic heart disease.

The ethnic variation in rates of mortality attributed to symptoms,

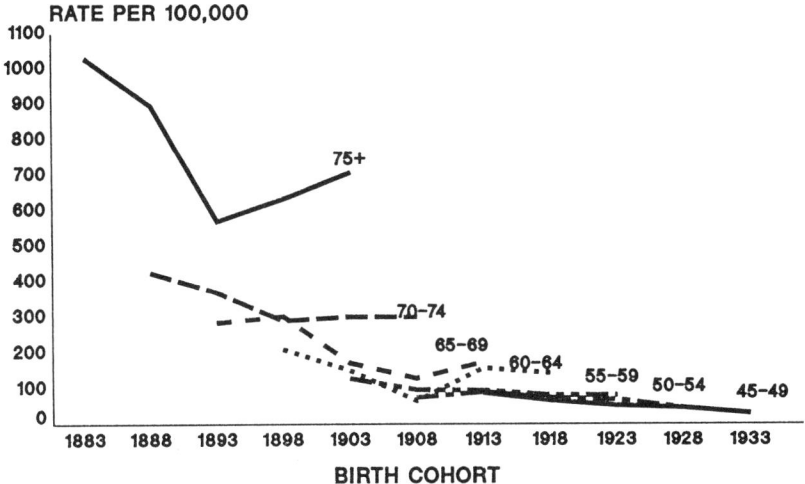

Figure 11.3. *Mortality from symptoms, signs, and ill-defined conditions among Hispanic males in New Mexico, by 5-year birth cohort.*

signs, and ill-defined conditions reflects the socioeconomic differences among New Mexico's American Indian, Hispanic, and non-Hispanic white populations. Other states with depressed economies and high proportions of minorities also show elevated mortality rates from this category (Table 11.1). This observation is particularly apparent in the south-central states with large minority (especially black) populations. In the Southwest, the population of Texas, which ranked seventh in the U.S. in mortality rates attributed to symptoms, signs, and ill-defined conditions in 1980, had a high proportion of both blacks (12%) and Hispanics (21%). We surmise that the disadvantaged minorities in these states, as in New Mexico, contribute disproportionately to mortality rates assigned to "cause of death unknown" codes.

Lack of health insurance for a substantial proportion of New Mexicans influences health care access and utilization. At present, 20% to 25% of New Mexicans have no health insurance, compared with 10% to 13% nationwide (Bennett and Mantlo 1988). In addition, rural residents and Hispanics in New Mexico are also less likely to have health

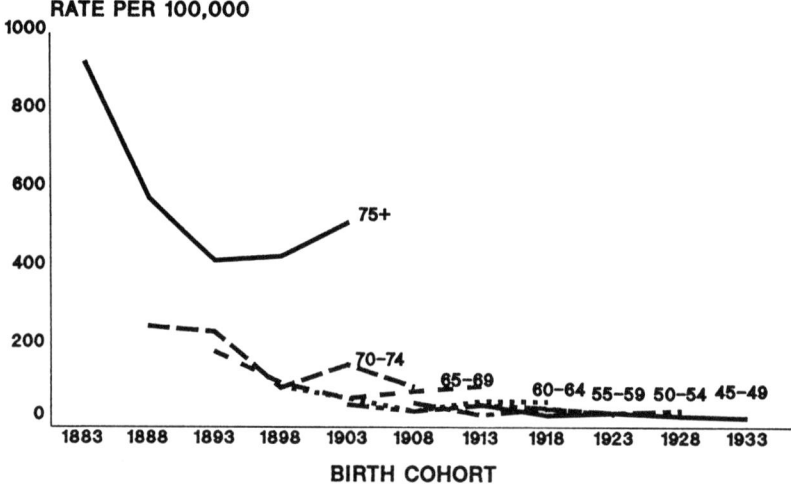

Figure 11.4. *Mortality from symptoms, signs, and ill-defined conditions among Hispanic females in New Mexico, by 5-year birth cohort.*

insurance than are urban residents and non-Hispanic whites (Bennett and Mantlo 1988). Statistics show that in New Mexico, Hispanics are twice as likely as non-Hispanics to be without health insurance (33% compared with 15%) (Bennett and Mantlo 1988). Since uninsured individuals use health services less frequently than insured persons (Dutton 1986; Bazzoli 1986), the large numbers of uninsured residents in the state are less likely to have consistent medical attention for chronic conditions that may lead to death. In the absence of autopsy, the lack of physician familiarity with an uninsured decedent's health status may commonly result in the assignment of death to the category of symptoms, signs, and ill-defined conditions.

New Mexico's geography may also exert an influence on health care availability. The lack of hospitals and clinics in some remote parts of the state constitutes a geographic barrier to easy access to health care (State of New Mexico 1985). In addition, physical barriers to travel—such as unpaved rural roads that become impassable during certain seasons—

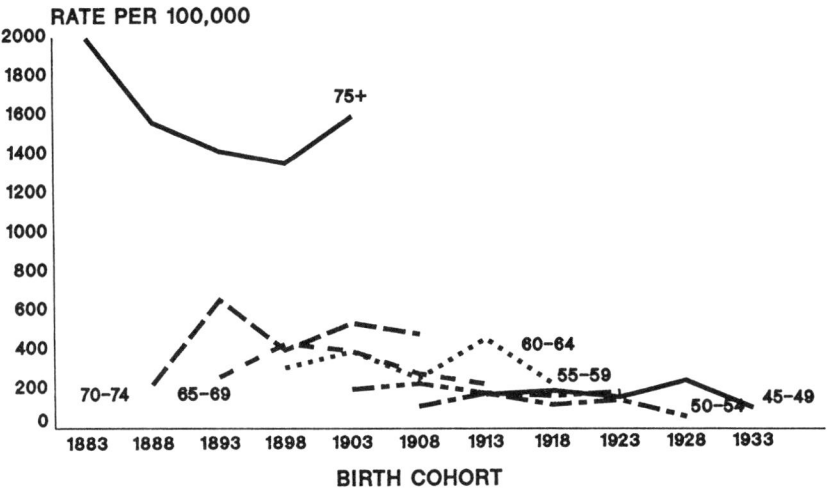

Figure 11.5. *Mortality from symptoms, signs, and ill-defined conditions among American Indian males in New Mexico, by 5-year birth cohort.*

provide another obstacle to obtaining health care, especially for the Navajo, many of whom live in remote areas (Williams 1987). Nevertheless, despite the potential influences of geography on health care access and utilization in New Mexico, we observed no differences between urban and rural dwellers in mortality rates ascribed to symptoms, signs, and ill-defined conditions.

The use of traditional methods of healing among American Indians and Hispanics may also increase the assignation of deaths to this category if people using the traditional healers avoid modern conventional medical care altogether. Among American Indians in the Southwest, traditional healers or medicine men continue to play a central role in the medical care of many ill persons (Ortiz 1979, 1983). For American Indians who use traditional healers exclusively, and who have died while under the care of a traditional healer, we surmise that deaths are more likely to be assigned eventually to the category symptoms, signs, and ill-defined conditions. Similarly, Hispanics who seek care from *curanderos* or *curan-*

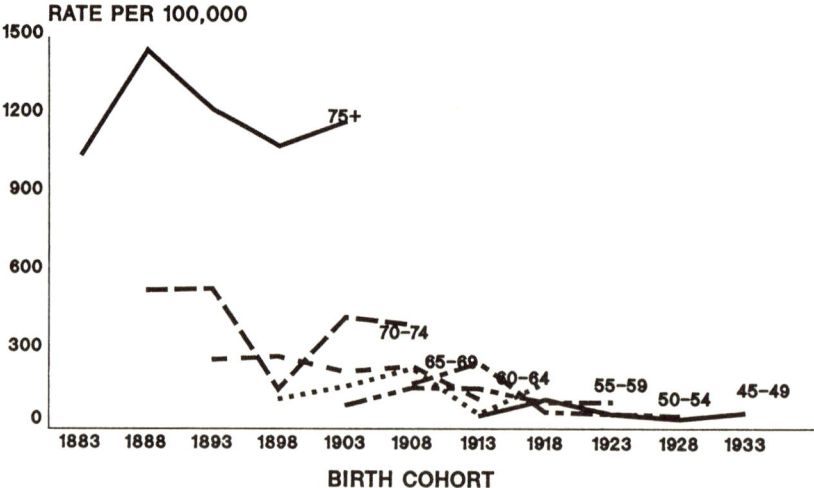

Figure 11.6. *Mortality from symptoms, signs, and ill-defined conditions among American Indian females in New Mexico, by 5-year birth cohort.*

deras, or traditional folk healers in New Mexico (Maduro 1983; Scheper-Hughes and Stewart 1983), and who die while under the care of such healers, may also have increased likelihood of attribution of death to this category.

The State Office of the Medical Investigator (OMI) is responsible for investigating all deaths that occur statewide in persons who are not under the care of an attending physician. The OMI was established in 1974; before that time, county coroners were primarily responsible for coding of death certificates and for performing autopsies. The OMI, however, does not have jurisdiction to investigate American Indian deaths that occur on reservation lands. Thus, the OMI can establish cause of death through autopsy for many Hispanics and non-Hispanic whites who die unattended by a physician, while many American Indian deaths remain uninvestigated, and fewer autopsies on American Indians are performed to establish cause of death. This lack of legal jurisdiction to perform autopsies on American Indian decedents may, therefore, further contribute

Table 11.3

Variation in ischemic heart disease mortality rates* in New Mexicans, adjusted by the addition of mortality for symptoms, signs, and ill-defined conditions, 1978 through 1982

Ethnic Group	IHD[a] deaths No. cases/(rate)	SSI[b] deaths No. cases/(rate)	IHD + 25% SSI deaths[c] No. cases/(rate)	IHD + 50% SSI deaths[c] No. cases/(rate)	IHD + 100% SSI deaths[c] No. cases/(rate)
Males					
Non-Hispanic white	3,727 (231.3)	792 (49.2)	3,925 (243.6)	4,123 (255.9)	4,519 (280.5)
Hispanic	1,133 (159.8)	452 (58.3)	1,246 (174.4)	1,359 (188.9)	1,585 (218.1)
American Indian	94 (76.6)	169 (115.6)	136 (105.5)	179 (134.4)	263 (192.3)
Females					
Non-Hispanic white	2,464 (109.8)	582 (27.9)	2,610 (116.8)	2,755 (123.8)	3,046 (137.7)
Hispanic	738 (91.6)	264 (30.9)	804 (99.3)	870 (107.0)	1,002 (122.5)
American Indian	36 (28.3)	123 (81.7)	67 (48.7)	98 (69.1)	159 (110.0)

*Age-adjusted rates per 100,000 (adjusted to 1970 U.S. population).
[a]Ischemic heart disease.
[b]Symptoms, signs, and ill-defined conditions.
[c]Ischemic heart disease deaths added to deaths from symptoms, signs, and ill-defined conditions.

Table 11.4

Variation in ischemic heart disease mortality rates* in elderly New Mexicans, adjusted by the addition of mortality from symptoms, signs, and ill-defined conditions, 1978 through 1982

Ethnic Group	IHD[a] deaths No. cases/(rate)	SSI[b] deaths No. cases/(rate)	IHD + 25% SSI deaths[c] No. cases/(rate)	IHD + 50% SSI deaths[c] No. cases/(rate)	IHD + 100% SSI deaths[c] No. cases/(rate)
Males					
Non-Hispanic white	1,405 (2,797.5)	246 (489.8)	1,467 (2,919.9)	1,529 (3,042.4)	1,651 (3,287.3)
Hispanic	505 (1,996.4)	177 (699.7)	549 (2,171.3)	594 (2,346.2)	682 (2,698.1)
American Indian	30 (673.6)	70 (1,571.6)	48 (1,066.5)	65 (1,459.4)	100 (2,245.2)
Females					
Non-Hispanic white	1,649 (1,905.5)	318 (367.4)	1,729 (1,997.3)	1,808 (2,089.2)	1,967 (2,272.9)
Hispanic	449 (1,499.2)	151 (504.1)	543 (1,812.1)	581 (1,938.2)	656 (2,190.3)
American Indian	21 (469.1)	52 (1,161.4)	34 (759.4)	47 (1,049.8)	73 (1,630.6)

* Age-specific rates per 100,000 for persons 75 years old and above.
[a] Ischemic heart disease.
[b] Symptoms, signs, and ill-defined conditions.
[c] Ischemic heart disease deaths added to deaths from symptoms, signs, and ill-defined conditions.

to the assignment of death to symptoms, signs, and ill-defined conditions among members of that ethnic group. On the other hand, the OMI also assigns cases under its jurisdiction to the category of symptoms, signs, and ill-defined conditions. From 1974 through 1982, the OMI commonly used ICD codes for the elderly deceased that reflected death from "natural causes" (Patricia McFeeley, M.D., personal communication 1988). The ICD codes associated with natural causes of death are included within the category of symptoms, signs, and ill-defined conditions. This practice probably explains the age-specific increases in death rates assigned to this category among the elderly deceased (especially Hispanics and non-Hispanic whites) beginning in the mid-1970's (Figures 11.1 through 11.4).

Using ischemic heart disease as an example, we showed the extent of bias that can potentially be introduced into death certificate-based mortality studies (Tables 11.3 and 11.4). Mortality rates from ischemic heart disease were increased substantially upon addition of deaths from symptoms, signs, and ill-defined conditions to ischemic heart disease deaths. Furthermore, the data indicate that for New Mexico, the extent of bias varies among ethnic groups for both age-adjusted and age-specific ischemic heart disease mortality rates. In other chapters, we reported strong ethnic differences in New Mexico in mortality rates from various diseases. Researchers should consider that cause-specific mortality rates (especially for chronic diseases) may be strongly influenced by the numbers of deaths that are included in the category of symptoms, signs, and ill-defined conditions.

Summary

Mortality rates attributed to symptoms, signs, and ill-defined conditions are high in all three major ethnic groups in New Mexico. The mortality rates attributed to this category exceeded the national rates for blacks and for whites in each of the state's major ethnic groups. We suggest that the mortality rate for deaths attributed to this category may be a potential indicator of health services access and use, and that categorization of cause of death from this category may also strongly affect cause-specific mortality rates in minority populations in this state and throughout the U.S.

REFERENCES

Bazzoli, G. J. 1986. Health care for the indigent: overview of critical issues. *Health Serv.Res.* 21:353–393.

Becker, T. M., C. L. Wiggins, C. R. Key, and J. M. Samet. 1988. Ischemic heart disease mortality in Hispanics, American Indians, and non-Hispanic whites in New Mexico, 1958–1982. *Circulation* 78:302–309.

———. 1989a. Ethnic differences in mortality from acute rheumatic fever and chronic rheumatic heart disease in New Mexico, 1958–82. *West.J.Med.* 150:46–50.

———. 1989b. Symptoms, signs, and ill-defined conditions: a leading cause of death among minorities. *Am.J.Epidemiol.* 131:664–668.

Bennett, M., and E. J. Mantlo. 1988. *New Mexico resources registry, statistical summary 1986–1987.* Albuquerque, NM: University of New Mexico Medical Center.

Dutton, D. B. 1986. Social class, health, and illness. In *Application of social science to clinical medicine and health policy,* edited by L. H. Aiken and D. Mechanic. New Brunswick, NJ: Rutgers University Press.

Key, C. R. 1981. *Cancer incidence and mortality in New Mexico, 1973–77. Surveillance, epidemiology, and end results: incidence mortality data, 1973–1977.* National Cancer Institute Monograph No. 57. Washington, DC: U.S. Department of Health and Human Services.

Maduro, R. 1983. *Curanderismo* and latino views of disease and curing. *West.J. Med.* 139:863–874.

Ortiz, A. ed. 1979. *Handbook of North American Indians.* Vol. 9, *Southwest.* Smithsonian Institution. Washington, DC: U.S. Government Printing Office.

———. 1983. *Handbook of North American Indians.* Vol. 10, *Southwest.* Smithsonian Institution. Washington, DC: U.S. Government Printing Office.

Samet, J. M., C. R. Key, D. M. Kutvirt, and C. L. Wiggins. 1980. Respiratory disease mortality in New Mexico's American Indians and Hispanics. *Am.J. Public Health* 70:492–497.

Samet, J. M., C. L. Wiggins, C. R. Key, and T. M. Becker. 1988. Mortality from lung cancer and chronic obstructive pulmonary disease in New Mexico, 1958–82. *Am.J.Public Health* 78:1182–1186.

Scheper-Hughes, N., and D. Stewart. 1983. *Curanderismo* in Taos County, New Mexico—possible case of anthropological romanticism. *West.J.Med.* 139:875–884.

State of New Mexico 1985. *Report of the New Mexico Health Care Cost and Access Commission 1985–86.* Santa Fe, NM: New Mexico Health Care Cost and Access Commission. 1985:1–51.

U.S. Bureau of the Census. 1981. *Census of the population, 1980. General population characteristics.* Final report PC80-1-B33, New Mexico. Washington, DC: U.S. Government Printing Office.

U.S. Department of Health and Human Services. 1982. *Vital statistics of the United States.* Vol. II, *Mortality,* Part A. DHHS Publication No. 86-1122. Washington, DC: U.S. Government Printing Office.

Wiggins, C. L., T. M. Becker, C. R. Key, and J. M. Samet. 1989. Stomach cancer among New Mexico's American Indians, Hispanics, and non-Hispanic whites. *Cancer Res.* 49:1595–1599.

Williams, R. 1987. Meningitis and unpaved roads. *Soc.Sci.Med.* 24:109–115.
World Health Organization. 1957. *Manual of the International Statistical Classification of Diseases, Injuries, and Causes of Death.* Based on the recommendations of the Seventh Revision Conference, 1955. Geneva, Switzerland: WHO.

CHAPTER 12

Summary

Thomas M. Becker

The preceding chapters show the variation in cause-specific mortality among the Hispanics, American Indians, and non-Hispanic whites in New Mexico, with striking ethnic- and sex-specific differences in the mortality rates apparent for many causes of death. Although we recognize the problems inherent in analyses of mortality data, we have demonstrated that such data can show general trends in cause-specific mortality, and so provide important information for public health planning. The background information on ethnic-specific differences in mortality in these data has already led to the development of some targeted intervention strategies to reduce infectious or chronic disease mortality rates. For the reader whose particular interest is not public health, the monograph also provides background data for further etiologic research in geographic medicine. Social and behavioral scientists may also find our analyses useful as they seek ethnic-specific data to support scholarly endeavors or requests for grant support for etiologic/intervention studies.

An updated analysis of the New Mexico Vital Records data will be made by this research group after several more years of data have been compiled. At that time, we will determine whether the decreasing mortality from infectious causes has continued, and will also examine the direction of currently evolving mortality trends for chronic diseases. We believe the recent advances in medical therapy, changing lifestyles, and the emerging importance of certain causes of death, such as AIDS, will result in changes in the patterns of cause-specific mortality. Changes in medical economics—such as cost-containment strategies—as well as the changing prevalence of risk factors for certain infectious and chronic diseases could also influence future mortality statistics in this state. Future investigations based on mortality data compiled since 1982 (the last year included in this study) must consider the many changes in behavior, medical care, and public health policies over the past 10 years.

The data up until the year 1982 of this monograph can be supplemented by the yearly reports published by the New Mexico Bureau of

Vital Statistics. Although such summaries usually lag two to three years behind the current calendar year, they are extremely useful sources of information in ethnic- and cause-specific mortality, and also give ethnic-specific data on the incidence of specific infections and certain chronic diseases. These annual published reports are available to public health officials and scholars by contacting Mr. Anthony Ortiz, Bureau of Vital Statistics, Public Health Department, Santa Fe, NM 87502.

The appendix to this volume contains computer-generated tables of age-adjusted mortality rates for specific causes of death. These tables show mortality rates for 5-year periods beginning in 1958 through 1982 and are organized by sex and by ethnic group. The data in these tables do not include adjustments for comparability when ICD mortality codes changed among the three ICD revisions used over the 25-year span of the data. These figures should be useful to scholars or researchers interested in diseases that we have not discussed in the preceding chapters.

APPENDIX

Average Annual Age-Adjusted Mortality Rates for 73 Causes, 1958–1982, New Mexico

AVG ANNUAL AGE-ADJ (1970 US STANDARD) MORTALITY RATES/100,000
NEW MEXICO RESIDENTS, 1958-82, BY ETHNICITY, SEX, AND CAUSE

ETHNIC TOTAL
AND SEX MALE

	YEAR_01				
	1958-62	1963-67	1968-72	1973-77	1978-82
	AGE_RATE	AGE_RATE	AGE_RATE	AGE_RATE	AGE_RATE
	SUM	SUM	SUM	SUM	SUM
SITE					
ALL SITES	1051.3	1035.8	1100.6	1060.0	968.8
INF & PARA DIS	28.8	22.5	14.0	11.9	7.5
TUBERCULOSIS	13.4	9.6	5.4	3.7	1.7
INF & PARASIT	15.4	12.9	8.5	8.1	5.8
TOTAL CANCER	128.3	131.4	150.4	160.6	185.9
BUC CAV & PHAR	2.3	3.3	3.6	3.5	3.7
ESOPHAGUS	2.3	2.2	3.2	2.4	3.1
STOMACH	19.5	12.2	12.1	9.5	9.5
COLON	8.6	9.3	12.4	14.4	16.0
RECTUM	3.9	2.5	3.5	3.1	3.6
LIVER & BIL	7.0	5.8	3.7	3.3	6.1
PANCREAS	6.8	9.6	9.6	9.9	10.7
LARYNX	1.5	1.4	1.6	1.6	1.9
TR, BR, & LUNG	22.5	27.1	37.4	43.7	50.9
OTHER RESPIR	0.4	0.2	0.3	0.3	0.1
BREAST	0.0	0.1	0.2	0.2	0.7
CERVIX	0.0	0.0	0.0	0.0	0.0
CORPUS UTERI	0.0	0.0	0.0	0.0	0.0
OTHER UTERUS	0.0	0.0	0.0	0.0	0.0
OVARY	0.0	0.0	0.0	0.0	0.0

(CONTINUED)

Source: Vital Statistics Bureau, New Mexico Health and Environment Department, Santa Fe, New Mexico.

MORTALITY RATES

AVG ANNUAL AGE-ADJ (1970 US STANDARD) MORTALITY RATES/100,000
NEW MEXICO RESIDENTS, 1958-82, BY ETHNICITY, SEX, AND CAUSE

ETHNIC TOTAL
AND SEX MALE

	YEAR_01				
	1958-62	1963-67	1968-72	1973-77	1978-82
	AGE_RATE	AGE_RATE	AGE_RATE	AGE_RATE	AGE_RATE
	SUM	SUM	SUM	SUM	SUM
SITE					
OTH FEM GEN	0.0	0.0	0.0	0.0	0.0
PROSTATE	15.6	15.0	18.1	18.1	23.4
TESTIS	0.7	0.5	0.7	0.4	0.3
OTH MALE GEN	0.3	0.2	0.3	0.1	0.3
KIDNEY	3.7	3.1	3.4	4.1	3.8
BLADDER	3.2	3.5	4.5	4.7	5.6
OTH URINARY	0.1	0.0	0.1	0.0	0.1
MELANOMA SKIN	0.8	1.4	1.7	2.0	2.1
OTHER SKIN	1.6	0.8	0.8	1.3	0.7
BRAIN	2.6	3.6	3.2	4.9	5.0
THYROID	0.4	0.4	0.3	0.3	0.3
BONE	0.9	1.6	1.1	0.8	0.7
LYMPH & RETIC	2.7	3.1	3.1	1.4	1.7
HODG LYMPH	1.2	2.2	1.9	1.4	0.9
LEUKEMIAS	6.2	8.2	6.2	7.2	7.8
OTH LYM & HEM	2.2	2.4	2.4	4.3	6.1
OTHER CANCER	10.0	10.6	13.6	16.4	19.5
OTH BRAIN CA	1.2	1.4	0.9	0.8	0.2
ALCOHOLISM	3.1	4.1	6.2	19.1	21.3
DIABETES	11.5	13.8	17.2	15.7	21.1

(CONTINUED)

AVG ANNUAL AGE-ADJ (1970 US STANDARD) MORTALITY RATES/100,000
NEW MEXICO RESIDENTS, 1958-82, BY ETHNICITY, SEX, AND CAUSE

ETHNIC TOTAL
AND SEX MALE

SITE	YEAR_01				
	1958-62	1963-67	1968-72	1973-77	1978-82
	AGE_RATE	AGE_RATE	AGE_RATE	AGE_RATE	AGE_RATE
	SUM	SUM	SUM	SUM	SUM
CIRCULATORY	419.5	414.0	456.7	404.1	325.6
RHEUM FEVER	0.3	0.2	0.4	0.5	0.3
CHRON RHM HRT	10.2	7.8	7.3	5.5	3.0
ISCHEMIC H D	220.4	232.9	272.8	242.9	182.3
HYPERTEN H D	17.0	14.5	5.7	2.5	5.2
HYPERTENSION	7.2	5.7	8.1	5.7	9.0
CEREBROVASC	89.1	76.8	90.4	73.1	52.0
OTH HRT & CIR	74.9	75.7	71.7	73.6	73.6
RESPIRATORY	82.8	90.1	104.3	105.9	92.3
ASTHMA	6.1	3.9	1.6	1.4	1.4
INFLUENZA	4.0	2.4	3.5	4.6	0.8
PNEUMONIA	44.2	40.4	49.6	47.9	27.7
CHR BRONCHI	1.8	3.6	2.8	1.2	0.6
EMPHYSEMA	10.3	26.8	29.3	19.3	12.1
COPD	0.0	0.0	2.3	22.3	38.7
OTH RESP DIS	16.2	12.8	14.7	8.8	10.6
PEPTIC ULCER	9.6	8.3	7.8	4.1	3.2
LIVER CIRRHO	15.5	18.9	27.4	26.2	20.4
NEPHRI -O	9.4	7.8	3.5	3.6	7.6
KIDNEY INFECT	4.2	4.6	3.5	1.7	0.8

(CONTINUED)

AVG ANNUAL AGE-ADJ (1970 US STANDARD) MORTALITY RATES/100,000 NEW MEXICO RESIDENTS, 1958-82, BY ETHNICITY, SEX, AND CAUSE

ETHNIC TOTAL
AND SEX MALE

	YEAR_01				
	1958-62	1963-67	1968-72	1973-77	1978-82
	AGE_RATE	AGE_RATE	AGE_RATE	AGE_RATE	AGE_RATE
SITE	SUM	SUM	SUM	SUM	SUM
PREGNANCY CMP	0.0	0.0	0.0	0.0	0.0
CONGENITAL AN	11.9	10.8	10.0	7.3	7.2
DIS INFANCY	46.9	38.9	25.8	16.1	11.8
SYMP, ILL-DEF	78.5	64.0	44.8	56.6	55.3
OTH DIS, NEC	49.8	55.1	50.1	50.7	54.6
TL EXTERNAL	149.7	149.4	177.1	174.8	153.2
MOTOR VEH ACC	60.3	58.4	70.3	69.0	60.9
OTHER ACC	61.7	62.2	64.4	54.5	40.0
SUICIDE	18.9	18.9	25.6	28.5	28.6
HOMICIDE	8.4	9.0	13.8	18.2	19.1
LEGAL INTRVNT	0.2	0.6	0.4	0.1	0.2

AVG ANNUAL AGE-ADJ (1970 US STANDARD) MORTALITY RATES/100,000
NEW MEXICO RESIDENTS, 1958-82, BY ETHNICITY, SEX, AND CAUSE

ETHNIC TOTAL
AND SEX FEMALE

	YEAR_01				
	1958-62	1963-67	1968-72	1973-77	1978-82
	AGE_RATE	AGE_RATE	AGE_RATE	AGE_RATE	AGE_RATE
	SUM	SUM	SUM	SUM	SUM
SITE					
ALL SITES	644.6	586.5	644.0	611.4	557.5
INF & PARA DIS	19.1	13.1	9.3	7.8	6.7
TUBERCULOSIS	7.6	3.9	1.8	1.6	1.1
INF & PARASIT	11.4	9.1	7.5	6.1	5.6
TOTAL CANCER	103.9	93.8	112.5	120.6	126.5
BUC CAV & PHAR	0.8	0.7	1.0	1.0	1.8
ESOPHAGUS	0.5	1.0	0.9	1.1	0.9
STOMACH	8.9	5.4	6.4	5.2	5.3
COLON	9.0	9.0	11.7	13.2	11.2
RECTUM	3.1	2.4	2.3	1.8	2.0
LIVER & BIL	8.3	5.3	4.5	4.7	4.9
PANCREAS	5.3	5.2	6.1	7.1	7.1
LARYNX	0.2	0.0	0.3	0.3	0.2
TR, BR, & LUNG	4.4	6.1	10.7	15.4	16.7
OTHER RESPIR	0.1	0.1	0.0	0.1	0.0
BREAST	16.5	16.7	20.3	19.3	24.0
CERVIX	8.0	6.6	5.7	5.1	3.0
CORPUS UTERI	0.4	0.6	1.2	1.5	1.7
OTHER UTERUS	3.8	2.5	2.5	1.6	1.6
OVARY	6.5	5.4	7.1	7.1	6.6

(CONTINUED)

MORTALITY RATES

AVG ANNUAL AGE-ADJ (1970 US STANDARD) MORTALITY RATES/100,000
NEW MEXICO RESIDENTS, 1958-82, BY ETHNICITY, SEX, AND CAUSE

ETHNIC TOTAL
AND SEX FEMALE

	YEAR_01				
	1958-62	1963-67	1968-72	1973-77	1978-82
	AGE_RATE	AGE_RATE	AGE_RATE	AGE_RATE	AGE_RATE
	SUM	SUM	SUM	SUM	SUM
SITE					
OTH FEM GEN	1.0	0.7	0.7	0.9	0.8
PROSTATE	0.0	0.0	0.0	0.0	0.0
TESTIS	0.0	0.0	0.0	0.0	0.0
OTH MALE GEN	0.0	0.0	0.0	0.0	0.0
KIDNEY	1.6	1.4	1.8	1.7	1.7
BLADDER	1.7	1.2	1.4	1.6	1.7
OTH URINARY	0.0	0.1	0.0	0.1	0.2
MELANOMA SKIN	1.1	0.9	1.0	1.2	1.6
OTHER SKIN	0.1	0.4	0.5	0.3	0.3
BRAIN	1.9	2.8	2.3	2.9	2.8
THYROID	0.6	0.3	0.5	0.5	0.5
BONE	0.7	0.6	0.4	0.5	0.5
LYMPH & RETIC	1.9	1.7	1.8	1.2	1.5
HODG LYMPH	1.0	0.9	1.0	0.8	0.4
LEUKEMIAS	4.4	5.1	4.5	4.0	5.3
OTH LYM & HEM	1.4	1.1	2.5	3.1	4.0
OTHER CANCER	9.4	8.2	11.9	16.0	16.6
OTH BRAIN CA	1.8	1.2	1.3	1.1	0.5
ALCOHOLISM	0.6	1.3	1.0	4.5	5.3
DIABETES	13.8	12.4	17.1	16.1	19.3

(CONTINUED)

AVG ANNUAL AGE-ADJ (1970 US STANDARD) MORTALITY RATES/100,000
NEW MEXICO RESIDENTS, 1958-82, BY ETHNICITY, SEX, AND CAUSE

ETHNIC TOTAL
AND SEX FEMALE

	YEAR_01				
	1958-62	1963-67	1968-72	1973-77	1978-82
	AGE_RATE	AGE_RATE	AGE_RATE	AGE_RATE	AGE_RATE
	SUM	SUM	SUM	SUM	SUM
SITE					
CIRCULATORY	267.6	239.1	279.1	249.6	202.8
RHEUM FEVER	0.4	0.2	0.4	0.5	0.7
CHRON RHM HRT	12.4	9.3	6.4	4.5	3.3
ISCHEMIC H D	105.7	101.1	136.2	118.5	92.0
HYPERTEN H D	19.5	14.9	4.4	2.1	5.0
HYPERTENSION	5.7	4.5	7.1	5.3	7.3
CEREBROVASC	70.6	59.9	76.2	69.2	46.6
OTH HRT & CIR	53.0	49.0	48.1	49.3	47.5
RESPIRATORY	44.6	42.1	51.6	51.2	44.5
ASTHMA	1.9	1.8	1.3	1.1	1.9
INFLUENZA	3.1	1.8	2.6	3.7	0.6
PNEUMONIA	28.3	25.1	31.5	28.9	17.9
CHR BRONCHI	0.5	1.0	0.9	0.3	0.0
EMPHYSEMA	1.3	3.6	5.9	4.4	4.3
COPD	0.0	0.0	0.6	7.5	14.9
OTH RESP DIS	9.2	8.6	8.5	4.9	4.6
PEPTIC ULCER	3.7	3.8	3.3	2.5	2.2
LIVER CIRRHO	8.1	8.4	12.0	10.2	8.1
NEPHRI -O	6.4	6.0	2.9	2.9	4.6
KIDNEY INFECT	2.9	4.6	4.0	1.5	0.6

(CONTINUED)

MORTALITY RATES

AVG ANNUAL AGE-ADJ (1970 US STANDARD) MORTALITY RATES/100,000
NEW MEXICO RESIDENTS, 1958-82, BY ETHNICITY, SEX, AND CAUSE

ETHNIC TOTAL
AND SEX FEMALE

	YEAR_01				
	1958-62	1963-67	1968-72	1973-77	1978-82
	AGE_RATE	AGE_RATE	AGE_RATE	AGE_RATE	AGE_RATE
	SUM	SUM	SUM	SUM	SUM
SITE					
PREGNANCY CMP	0.8	0.6	0.7	0.5	0.5
CONGENITAL AN	9.5	9.3	7.6	6.7	4.9
DIS INFANCY	35.7	29.6	18.7	11.2	8.6
SYMP, ILL-DEF	37.7	30.6	24.4	28.6	30.5
OTH DIS, NEC	40.0	40.4	38.5	38.7	42.9
TL EXTERNAL	47.5	49.4	59.3	56.9	48.3
MOTOR VEH ACC	18.4	18.7	24.0	22.2	19.4
OTHER ACC	21.3	23.1	24.1	18.5	14.1
SUICIDE	4.6	4.6	6.4	8.7	7.6
HOMICIDE	3.0	2.9	4.0	5.6	5.1
LEGAL INTRVNT	0.0	0.0	0.0	0.0	0.0

AVG ANNUAL AGE-ADJ (1970 US STANDARD) MORTALITY RATES/100,000
NEW MEXICO RESIDENTS, 1958-82, BY ETHNICITY, SEX, AND CAUSE

ETHNIC WHITE
AND SEX MALE

	YEAR_01				
	1958-62	1963-67	1968-72	1973-77	1978-82
	AGE_RATE	AGE_RATE	AGE_RATE	AGE_RATE	AGE_RATE
	SUM	SUM	SUM	SUM	SUM
SITE					
ALL SITES	1044.0	1026.8	1081.0	1030.7	954.4
INF & PARA DIS	24.1	17.7	10.8	9.6	6.5
TUBERCULOSIS	11.4	7.9	4.1	2.5	1.3
INF & PARASIT	12.7	9.8	6.7	7.0	5.2
TOTAL CANCER	131.5	134.1	152.8	163.5	189.3
BUC CAV & PHAR	2.4	3.4	3.6	3.6	3.8
ESOPHAGUS	2.2	2.2	3.2	2.5	3.1
STOMACH	20.0	12.1	11.8	8.9	9.2
COLON	9.0	9.8	13.0	15.0	16.7
RECTUM	4.1	2.5	3.5	3.2	3.7
LIVER & BIL	7.0	5.6	3.5	3.1	5.5
PANCREAS	6.9	9.8	9.8	10.3	11.0
LARYNX	1.6	1.4	1.8	1.6	1.9
TR, BR, & LUNG	23.5	28.2	38.8	45.1	52.6
OTHER RESPIR	0.4	0.2	0.3	0.3	0.1
BREAST	0.0	0.1	0.2	0.2	0.7
CERVIX	0.0	0.0	0.0	0.0	0.0
CORPUS UTERI	0.0	0.0	0.0	0.0	0.0
OTHER UTERUS	0.0	0.0	0.0	0.0	0.0
OVARY	0.0	0.0	0.0	0.0	0.0

(CONTINUED)

MORTALITY RATES

AVG ANNUAL AGE-ADJ (1970 US STANDARD) MORTALITY RATES/100,000
NEW MEXICO RESIDENTS, 1958-82, BY ETHNICITY, SEX, AND CAUSE

ETHNIC WHITE
AND SEX MALE

	YEAR_01				
	1958-62	1963-67	1968-72	1973-77	1978-82
	AGE_RATE	AGE_RATE	AGE_RATE	AGE_RATE	AGE_RATE
SITE	SUM	SUM	SUM	SUM	SUM
OTH FEM GEN	0.0	0.0	0.0	0.0	0.0
PROSTATE	15.9	15.2	18.0	18.0	23.6
TESTIS	0.7	0.5	0.7	0.4	0.3
OTH MALE GEN	0.2	0.2	0.4	0.1	0.2
KIDNEY	3.5	3.0	3.4	4.0	4.0
BLADDER	3.4	3.6	4.6	5.0	5.9
OTH URINARY	0.1	0.1	0.1	0.0	0.1
MELANOMA SKIN	0.8	1.5	1.8	2.2	2.3
OTHER SKIN	1.6	0.9	0.9	1.4	0.8
BRAIN	2.7	3.8	3.1	5.1	5.1
THYROID	0.5	0.4	0.2	0.3	0.3
BONE	0.9	1.6	1.1	0.8	0.7
LYMPH & RETIC	2.7	3.1	3.1	1.4	1.8
HODG LYMPH	1.3	2.4	2.0	1.4	0.9
LEUKEMIAS	6.4	8.5	6.5	7.4	8.1
OTH LYM & HEM	2.3	2.5	2.4	4.2	6.2
OTHER CANCER	9.8	10.3	13.6	16.5	19.3
OTH BRAIN CA	1.3	1.3	0.9	0.9	0.2
ALCOHOLISM	2.6	3.8	4.7	13.8	17.5
DIABETES	11.3	14.1	16.6	15.2	21.0

(CONTINUED)

AVG ANNUAL AGE-ADJ (1970 US STANDARD) MORTALITY RATES/100,000
NEW MEXICO RESIDENTS, 1958-82, BY ETHNICITY, SEX, AND CAUSE

ETHNIC WHITE
AND SEX MALE

	YEAR_01				
	1958-62	1963-67	1968-72	1973-77	1978-82
	AGE_RATE	AGE_RATE	AGE_RATE	AGE_RATE	AGE_RATE
	SUM	SUM	SUM	SUM	SUM
SITE					
CIRCULATORY	430.9	426.8	468.2	412.5	332.8
RHEUM FEVER	0.3	0.2	0.4	0.4	0.3
CHRON RHM HRT	10.3	7.9	6.7	5.2	3.2
ISCHEMIC H D	228.8	243.3	283.8	251.6	188.6
HYPERTEN H D	17.0	14.8	5.9	2.5	5.4
HYPERTENSION	7.0	5.7	8.5	5.7	8.9
CEREBROVASC	90.6	77.5	90.2	73.3	52.8
OTH HRT & CIR	76.6	77.0	72.4	73.6	73.4
RESPIRATORY	80.9	90.1	102.9	105.0	92.9
ASTHMA	6.3	4.2	1.6	1.5	1.4
INFLUENZA	3.7	2.4	3.6	4.5	0.9
PNEUMONIA	41.6	38.4	46.8	45.7	26.7
CHR BRONCHI	1.9	3.8	3.0	1.2	0.7
EMPHYSEMA	11.0	28.3	31.2	20.5	12.8
COPD	0.0	0.0	2.4	23.1	40.7
OTH RESP DIS	16.2	12.9	14.0	8.3	9.5
PEPTIC ULCER	10.1	8.8	8.3	4.2	3.3
LIVER CIRRHO	15.6	18.9	25.0	23.0	19.7
NEPHRI -O	9.1	7.2	3.2	3.2	7.3
KIDNEY INFECT	3.7	4.3	3.4	1.7	0.8

(CONTINUED)

MORTALITY RATES

AVG ANNUAL AGE-ADJ (1970 US STANDARD) MORTALITY RATES/100,000
NEW MEXICO RESIDENTS, 1958-82, BY ETHNICITY, SEX, AND CAUSE

ETHNIC WHITE
AND SEX MALE

	YEAR_01				
	1958-62	1963-67	1968-72	1973-77	1978-82
	AGE_RATE SUM	AGE_RATE SUM	AGE_RATE SUM	AGE_RATE SUM	AGE_RATE SUM
SITE					
PREGNANCY CMP	0.0	0.0	0.0	0.0	0.0
CONGENITAL AN	12.2	10.5	9.9	7.3	6.9
DIS INFANCY	47.0	39.0	25.6	15.8	11.4
SYMP, ILL-DEF	72.4	55.9	39.0	51.7	51.8
OTH DIS, NEC	48.7	53.9	47.7	47.8	53.1
TL EXTERNAL	141.9	139.7	161.3	154.7	139.1
MOTOR VEH ACC	56.5	54.7	62.5	58.6	54.2
OTHER ACC	59.3	57.5	59.1	48.9	35.6
SUICIDE	18.8	19.0	25.3	27.4	28.0
HOMICIDE	6.9	7.6	11.6	15.8	17.1
LEGAL INTRVNT	0.2	0.5	0.4	0.0	0.2

AVG ANNUAL AGE-ADJ (1970 US STANDARD) MORTALITY RATES/100,000
NEW MEXICO RESIDENTS, 1958-82, BY ETHNICITY, SEX, AND CAUSE

ETHNIC WHITE
AND SEX FEMALE

	YEAR_01				
	1958-62	1963-67	1968-72	1973-77	1978-82
	AGE_RATE	AGE_RATE	AGE_RATE	AGE_RATE	AGE_RATE
	SUM	SUM	SUM	SUM	SUM
SITE					
ALL SITES	637.9	570.9	628.0	599.3	551.7
INF & PARA DIS	15.4	9.1	7.1	6.2	6.1
TUBERCULOSIS	6.1	2.6	1.0	1.1	0.8
INF & PARASIT	9.3	6.5	6.1	5.0	5.3
TOTAL CANCER	105.3	94.6	114.3	122.2	128.3
BUC CAV & PHAR	0.8	0.8	1.1	1.1	1.8
ESOPHAGUS	0.5	0.9	0.9	1.1	1.0
STOMACH	9.1	5.3	6.5	5.4	5.2
COLON	9.2	9.4	12.4	13.6	11.5
RECTUM	3.2	2.5	2.4	1.8	2.1
LIVER & BIL	7.9	4.9	4.1	4.1	4.4
PANCREAS	4.9	5.3	6.0	6.9	7.1
LARYNX	0.2	0.0	0.3	0.3	0.3
TR, BR, & LUNG	4.5	6.3	11.1	16.1	17.2
OTHER RESPIR	0.2	0.1	0.0	0.1	0.0
BREAST	17.1	17.3	20.7	19.8	24.7
CERVIX	8.2	6.4	5.6	5.0	2.8
CORPUS UTERI	0.4	0.6	1.2	1.6	1.7
OTHER UTERUS	3.8	2.4	2.6	1.7	1.7
OVARY	6.4	5.6	7.4	7.3	6.9

(CONTINUED)

MORTALITY RATES

AVG ANNUAL AGE-ADJ (1970 US STANDARD) MORTALITY RATES/100,000
NEW MEXICO RESIDENTS, 1958-82, BY ETHNICITY, SEX, AND CAUSE

ETHNIC WHITE
AND SEX FEMALE

	YEAR_01				
	1958-62	1963-67	1968-72	1973-77	1978-82
	AGE_RATE	AGE_RATE	AGE_RATE	AGE_RATE	AGE_RATE
	SUM	SUM	SUM	SUM	SUM
SITE					
OTH FEM GEN	1.0	0.8	0.6	0.8	0.7
PROSTATE	0.0	0.0	0.0	0.0	0.0
TESTIS	0.0	0.0	0.0	0.0	0.0
OTH MALE GEN	0.0	0.0	0.0	0.0	0.0
KIDNEY	1.6	1.3	1.9	1.7	1.6
BLADDER	1.7	1.2	1.4	1.7	1.8
OTH URINARY	0.0	0.1	0.0	0.0	0.2
MELANOMA SKIN	1.1	0.9	1.0	1.3	1.7
OTHER SKIN	0.2	0.4	0.6	0.3	0.3
BRAIN	2.1	3.0	2.4	3.0	3.1
THYROID	0.7	0.2	0.6	0.5	0.5
BONE	0.7	0.7	0.3	0.5	0.5
LYMPH & RETIC	2.0	1.8	1.9	1.2	1.6
HODG LYMPH	1.1	0.9	1.0	0.9	0.4
LEUKEMIAS	4.7	5.5	4.8	4.1	5.6
OTH LYM & HEM	1.4	1.0	2.5	3.0	4.0
OTHER CANCER	9.4	7.6	11.5	15.7	16.3
OTH BRAIN CA	1.8	1.3	1.3	1.1	0.5
ALCOHOLISM	0.5	1.2	0.5	3.0	4.2
DIABETES	14.2	12.5	16.4	15.7	18.6

(CONTINUED)

**AVG ANNUAL AGE-ADJ (1970 US STANDARD) MORTALITY RATES/100,000
NEW MEXICO RESIDENTS, 1958-82, BY ETHNICITY, SEX, AND CAUSE**

ETHNIC WHITE
AND SEX FEMALE

	YEAR_01				
	1958-62	1963-67	1968-72	1973-77	1978-82
	AGE_RATE	AGE_RATE	AGE_RATE	AGE_RATE	AGE_RATE
	SUM	SUM	SUM	SUM	SUM
SITE					
CIRCULATORY	273.8	242.6	280.6	252.8	206.1
RHEUM FEVER	0.4	0.2	0.3	0.6	0.8
CHRON RHM HRT	12.7	9.5	6.2	4.2	3.2
ISCHEMIC H D	108.9	103.5	138.4	121.3	94.6
HYPERTEN H D	19.7	14.7	4.5	2.2	5.1
HYPERTENSION	5.6	4.4	6.9	5.3	7.4
CEREBROVASC	71.7	61.0	76.4	70.0	47.1
OTH HRT & CIR	54.6	49.0	47.6	49.1	47.5
RESPIRATORY	41.9	40.5	49.3	50.5	44.5
ASTHMA	2.0	1.9	1.3	1.1	1.9
INFLUENZA	2.9	1.7	2.6	3.8	0.6
PNEUMONIA	25.7	23.1	29.9	27.9	17.2
CHR BRONCHI	0.5	1.1	0.9	0.3	0.0
EMPHYSEMA	1.4	3.7	6.2	4.6	4.6
COPD	0.0	0.0	0.5	7.7	15.6
OTH RESP DIS	9.1	8.7	7.5	4.7	4.4
PEPTIC ULCER	3.8	3.9	3.5	2.5	2.2
LIVER CIRRHO	8.0	7.6	10.0	8.3	7.5
NEPHRI -O	6.1	5.4	2.4	2.6	3.9
KIDNEY INFECT	2.5	4.1	3.7	1.4	0.6

(CONTINUED)

MORTALITY RATES

AVG ANNUAL AGE-ADJ (1970 US STANDARD) MORTALITY RATES/100,000
NEW MEXICO RESIDENTS, 1958-82, BY ETHNICITY, SEX, AND CAUSE

ETHNIC WHITE
AND SEX FEMALE

	YEAR_01				
	1958-62	1963-67	1968-72	1973-77	1978-82
	AGE_RATE	AGE_RATE	AGE_RATE	AGE_RATE	AGE_RATE
	SUM	SUM	SUM	SUM	SUM
SITE					
PREGNANCY CMP	0.8	0.4	0.5	0.5	0.4
CONGENITAL AN	9.7	9.6	7.8	6.5	4.7
DIS INFANCY	35.7	29.6	18.3	11.0	8.9
SYMP, ILL-DEF	33.4	23.6	20.6	25.9	28.0
OTH DIS, NEC	38.6	38.3	36.7	36.2	41.7
TL EXTERNAL	45.6	45.7	54.2	52.1	44.7
MOTOR VEH ACC	17.4	17.0	20.7	19.1	16.6
OTHER ACC	20.8	21.6	22.9	17.7	13.0
SUICIDE	4.8	4.8	6.6	8.9	8.0
HOMICIDE	2.4	2.2	3.3	4.8	5.0
LEGAL INTRVNT	0.0	0.0	0.0	0.0	0.0

AVG ANNUAL AGE-ADJ (1970 US STANDARD) MORTALITY RATES/100,000
NEW MEXICO RESIDENTS, 1958-82, BY ETHNICITY, SEX, AND CAUSE

ETHNIC ANGLO
AND SEX MALE

	YEAR_01				
	1958-62	1963-67	1968-72	1973-77	1978-82
	AGE_RATE	AGE_RATE	AGE_RATE	AGE_RATE	AGE_RATE
SITE	SUM	SUM	SUM	SUM	SUM
ALL SITES	1086.8	1054.4	1097.2	1066.0	964.1
INF & PARA DIS	17.6	12.8	8.3	9.0	5.7
TUBERCULOSIS	9.8	6.8	3.6	2.0	0.7
INF & PARASIT	7.7	6.0	4.6	7.0	4.9
TOTAL CANCER	142.2	143.0	166.4	183.1	204.7
BUC CAV & PHAR	2.7	4.2	4.4	4.4	4.3
ESOPHAGUS	2.5	2.3	3.3	2.9	3.1
STOMACH	13.6	7.8	6.0	5.9	6.2
COLON	10.4	11.7	16.5	17.2	19.3
RECTUM	4.9	2.7	3.4	3.1	3.4
LIVER & BIL	6.6	4.3	3.1	2.4	4.4
PANCREAS	7.1	10.1	9.9	9.0	10.5
LARYNX	1.6	1.2	2.1	1.6	2.1
TR, BR, & LUNG	30.1	34.6	48.3	56.6	62.9
OTHER RESPIR	0.5	0.1	0.0	0.4	0.1
BREAST	0.0	0.1	0.4	0.4	1.0
CERVIX	0.0	0.0	0.0	0.0	0.0
CORPUS UTERI	0.0	0.0	0.0	0.0	0.0
OTHER UTERUS	0.0	0.0	0.0	0.0	0.0
OVARY	0.0	0.0	0.0	0.0	0.0

(CONTINUED)

MORTALITY RATES

AVG ANNUAL AGE-ADJ (1970 US STANDARD) MORTALITY RATES/100,000
NEW MEXICO RESIDENTS, 1958-82, BY ETHNICITY, SEX, AND CAUSE

ETHNIC ANGLO
AND SEX MALE

	YEAR_01				
	1958-62	1963-67	1968-72	1973-77	1978-82
	AGE_RATE	AGE_RATE	AGE_RATE	AGE_RATE	AGE_RATE
	SUM	SUM	SUM	SUM	SUM
SITE					
OTH FEM GEN	0.0	0.0	0.0	0.0	0.0
PROSTATE	18.6	15.9	18.4	19.8	25.4
TESTIS	0.7	0.3	0.5	0.6	0.3
OTH MALE GEN	0.1	0.1	0.1	0.1	0.2
KIDNEY	4.5	3.5	3.7	4.2	4.0
BLADDER	4.4	4.8	5.8	6.0	6.9
OTH URINARY	0.0	0.1	0.1	0.1	0.2
MELANOMA SKIN	1.0	2.2	2.3	3.2	3.2
OTHER SKIN	2.0	1.0	1.0	1.8	1.1
BRAIN	3.2	4.5	3.8	6.0	5.6
THYROID	0.5	0.3	0.2	0.3	0.3
BONE	0.8	1.4	1.1	0.9	0.8
LYMPH & RETIC	3.5	3.2	3.5	1.6	2.1
HODG LYMPH	1.5	2.9	2.1	1.5	0.8
LEUKEMIAS	7.8	9.4	7.8	8.5	8.9
OTH LYM & HEM	3.2	3.1	2.8	5.3	6.7
OTHER CANCER	9.4	10.0	14.7	18.1	19.6
OTH BRAIN CA	1.3	1.4	1.1	1.0	0.2
ALCOHOLISM	2.3	2.7	3.4	9.7	11.2
DIABETES	12.0	13.3	13.4	12.2	18.0

(CONTINUED)

AVG ANNUAL AGE-ADJ (1970 US STANDARD) MORTALITY RATES/100,000
NEW MEXICO RESIDENTS, 1958-82, BY ETHNICITY, SEX, AND CAUSE

ETHNIC ANGLO
AND SEX MALE

	YEAR_01				
	1958-62	1963-67	1968-72	1973-77	1978-82
	AGE_RATE	AGE_RATE	AGE_RATE	AGE_RATE	AGE_RATE
	SUM	SUM	SUM	SUM	SUM
SITE					
CIRCULATORY	486.1	461.5	507.3	454.6	356.5
RHEUM FEVER	0.3	0.2	0.5	0.3	0.2
CHRON RHM HRT	10.5	7.1	7.2	4.5	3.0
ISCHEMIC H D	273.7	280.2	315.0	282.5	208.4
HYPERTEN H D	16.5	13.2	5.1	2.3	5.7
HYPERTENSION	7.2	5.4	7.7	5.9	9.0
CEREBROVASC	95.0	78.8	94.6	77.5	54.7
OTH HRT & CIR	82.6	76.3	76.8	81.2	75.2
RESPIRATORY	80.6	96.7	108.6	112.3	99.4
ASTHMA	7.9	5.5	1.8	1.7	1.7
INFLUENZA	2.9	2.3	3.9	4.3	0.8
PNEUMONIA	35.0	34.5	41.0	42.3	23.2
CHR BRONCHI	2.3	5.0	4.0	1.5	0.9
EMPHYSEMA	14.6	36.8	40.9	26.8	15.9
COPD	0.0	0.0	3.0	27.9	47.6
OTH RESP DIS	17.6	12.5	13.7	7.5	9.0
PEPTIC ULCER	12.1	8.5	8.5	3.7	3.3
LIVER CIRRHO	13.5	15.0	14.4	14.3	13.8
NEPHRI -O	8.4	6.8	3.1	2.9	7.2
KIDNEY INFECT	3.3	3.9	2.9	1.8	0.7

(CONTINUED)

MORTALITY RATES

**AVG ANNUAL AGE-ADJ (1970 US STANDARD) MORTALITY RATES/100,000
NEW MEXICO RESIDENTS, 1958-82, BY ETHNICITY, SEX, AND CAUSE**

ETHNIC ANGLO
AND SEX MALE

	YEAR_01				
	1958-62	1963-67	1968-72	1973-77	1978-82
	AGE_RATE	AGE_RATE	AGE_RATE	AGE_RATE	AGE_RATE
	SUM	SUM	SUM	SUM	SUM
SITE					
PREGNANCY CMP	0.0	0.0	0.0	0.0	0.0
CONGENITAL AN	12.0	11.4	10.0	7.9	6.8
DIS INFANCY	47.8	43.5	27.6	17.3	12.5
SYMP, ILL-DEF	58.3	42.9	31.9	49.1	49.2
OTH DIS, NEC	49.1	49.7	45.9	45.6	48.2
TL EXTERNAL	139.3	140.6	143.9	140.8	126.1
MOTOR VEH ACC	51.1	50.1	53.0	49.3	49.1
OTHER ACC	60.3	61.3	53.6	48.2	34.3
SUICIDE	23.4	22.9	28.6	28.8	28.6
HOMICIDE	4.1	5.8	6.2	11.1	10.8
LEGAL INTRVNT	0.2	0.2	0.2	0.0	0.0

AVG ANNUAL AGE-ADJ (1970 US STANDARD) MORTALITY RATES/100,000
NEW MEXICO RESIDENTS, 1958-82, BY ETHNICITY, SEX, AND CAUSE

ETHNIC ANGLO
AND SEX FEMALE

	YEAR_01				
	1958-62	1963-67	1968-72	1973-77	1978-82
	AGE_RATE	AGE_RATE	AGE_RATE	AGE_RATE	AGE_RATE
	SUM	SUM	SUM	SUM	SUM
SITE					
ALL SITES	607.7	542.5	609.5	604.1	561.8
INF & PARA DIS	10.1	6.8	5.4	5.1	5.8
TUBERCULOSIS	3.9	1.7	0.4	0.6	0.6
INF & PARASIT	6.1	5.0	4.9	4.4	5.1
TOTAL CANCER	104.1	92.1	115.7	124.0	132.7
BUC CAV & PHAR	0.8	0.8	1.4	1.2	2.0
ESOPHAGUS	0.7	0.6	0.7	0.9	1.2
STOMACH	5.3	3.3	4.2	3.8	3.8
COLON	10.6	9.8	14.1	14.8	12.5
RECTUM	3.3	2.5	2.6	1.9	2.1
LIVER & BIL	5.8	3.0	2.4	2.1	3.0
PANCREAS	4.4	4.6	5.7	6.4	6.3
LARYNX	0.0	0.1	0.4	0.2	0.3
TR, BR, & LUNG	4.5	6.8	10.8	17.9	19.9
OTHER RESPIR	0.3	0.0	0.0	0.0	0.1
BREAST	20.3	19.6	24.0	22.1	26.8
CERVIX	7.0	5.0	4.5	4.0	2.2
CORPUS UTERI	0.2	0.5	1.3	1.8	1.8
OTHER UTERUS	3.9	2.4	2.2	1.7	1.9
OVARY	7.3	5.7	8.0	7.6	7.3

(CONTINUED)

MORTALITY RATES

AVG ANNUAL AGE-ADJ (1970 US STANDARD) MORTALITY RATES/100,000
NEW MEXICO RESIDENTS, 1958-82, BY ETHNICITY, SEX, AND CAUSE

ETHNIC ANGLO
AND SEX FEMALE

SITE	1958-62 AGE_RATE SUM	1963-67 AGE_RATE SUM	1968-72 AGE_RATE SUM	1973-77 AGE_RATE SUM	1978-82 AGE_RATE SUM
OTH FEM GEN	0.6	0.8	0.8	0.9	0.7
PROSTATE	0.0	0.0	0.0	0.0	0.0
TESTIS	0.0	0.0	0.0	0.0	0.0
OTH MALE GEN	0.0	0.0	0.0	0.0	0.0
KIDNEY	2.0	1.4	2.0	1.6	1.7
BLADDER	1.7	1.1	1.6	1.7	1.9
OTH URINARY	0.0	0.0	0.0	0.0	0.3
MELANOMA SKIN	1.5	1.1	1.4	1.6	2.3
OTHER SKIN	0.1	0.4	0.5	0.3	0.2
BRAIN	2.8	3.5	2.7	3.4	3.6
THYROID	0.3	0.0	0.7	0.5	0.2
BONE	0.7	0.6	0.3	0.6	0.5
LYMPH & RETIC	1.8	2.1	2.0	1.2	1.8
HODG LYMPH	1.6	1.0	0.9	0.8	0.4
LEUKEMIAS	5.6	5.8	5.0	4.8	6.1
OTH LYM & HEM	1.5	1.1	2.4	3.4	4.2
OTHER CANCER	8.0	7.0	11.6	15.3	16.4
OTH BRAIN CA	2.3	1.5	1.2	0.9	0.5
ALCOHOLISM	0.5	1.4	0.3	3.0	3.9
DIABETES	13.5	9.6	12.0	12.3	15.0

(CONTINUED)

APPENDIX

AVG ANNUAL AGE-ADJ (1970 US STANDARD) MORTALITY RATES/100,000 NEW MEXICO RESIDENTS, 1958-82, BY ETHNICITY, SEX, AND CAUSE

ETHNIC ANGLO
AND SEX FEMALE

	YEAR_01				
	1958-62	1963-67	1968-72	1973-77	1978-82
	AGE_RATE	AGE_RATE	AGE_RATE	AGE_RATE	AGE_RATE
SITE	SUM	SUM	SUM	SUM	SUM
CIRCULATORY	272.0	234.8	277.7	259.8	213.4
RHEUM FEVER	0.4	0.1	0.4	0.6	0.7
CHRON RHM HRT	10.6	8.5	5.7	4.0	3.2
ISCHEMIC H D	116.3	102.2	139.6	127.4	99.0
HYPERTEN H D	18.6	12.5	3.7	2.4	5.3
HYPERTENSION	5.1	3.7	5.3	5.1	7.0
CEREBROVASC	69.9	60.2	76.1	70.7	48.3
OTH HRT & CIR	50.8	47.3	46.6	49.2	49.6
RESPIRATORY	34.0	35.1	43.0	49.1	46.3
ASTHMA	2.5	2.5	1.5	1.5	2.2
INFLUENZA	2.9	1.2	1.7	3.6	0.7
PNEUMONIA	19.3	18.7	25.4	26.0	15.9
CHR BRONCHI	0.4	1.0	0.8	0.3	0.0
EMPHYSEMA	1.1	3.5	6.2	5.1	5.4
COPD	0.0	0.0	0.6	7.4	17.3
OTH RESP DIS	7.5	7.9	6.5	5.0	4.5
PEPTIC ULCER	3.7	3.4	3.7	2.6	2.4
LIVER CIRRHO	7.7	6.9	8.8	8.6	6.2
NEPHRI -O	4.6	4.0	1.7	1.9	3.6
KIDNEY INFECT	2.5	3.5	3.6	1.6	0.7

(CONTINUED)

MORTALITY RATES

AVG ANNUAL AGE-ADJ (1970 US STANDARD) MORTALITY RATES/100,000
NEW MEXICO RESIDENTS, 1958-82, BY ETHNICITY, SEX, AND CAUSE

ETHNIC ANGLO
AND SEX FEMALE

	YEAR_01				
	1958-62	1963-67	1968-72	1973-77	1978-82
	AGE_RATE	AGE_RATE	AGE_RATE	AGE_RATE	AGE_RATE
	SUM	SUM	SUM	SUM	SUM
SITE					
PREGNANCY CMP	0.2	0.4	0.3	0.3	0.2
CONGENITAL AN	10.4	10.3	8.6	6.4	4.7
DIS INFANCY	36.8	32.8	19.5	12.7	8.6
SYMP, ILL-DEF	18.9	16.8	17.7	23.9	27.9
OTH DIS, NEC	35.4	32.9	34.2	34.8	41.3
TL EXTERNAL	50.3	49.4	55.3	56.3	47.8
MOTOR VEH ACC	19.1	18.7	20.6	19.0	17.3
OTHER ACC	22.6	21.8	22.8	18.4	14.0
SUICIDE	6.5	6.7	8.2	11.7	8.9
HOMICIDE	1.9	2.0	3.4	5.3	5.1
LEGAL INTRVNT	0.0	0.0	0.0	0.0	0.0

AVG ANNUAL AGE-ADJ (1970 US STANDARD) MORTALITY RATES/100,000
NEW MEXICO RESIDENTS, 1958-82, BY ETHNICITY, SEX, AND CAUSE

ETHNIC HISPANIC
AND SEX MALE

	YEAR_01				
	1958-62	1963-67	1968-72	1973-77	1978-82
	AGE_RATE	AGE_RATE	AGE_RATE	AGE_RATE	AGE_RATE
	SUM	SUM	SUM	SUM	SUM
SITE					
ALL SITES	953.4	968.8	1036.5	951.3	922.2
INF & PARA DIS	33.1	24.9	14.9	10.5	7.7
TUBERCULOSIS	14.1	10.0	5.1	3.8	2.5
INF & PARASIT	19.0	14.9	9.7	6.7	5.1
TOTAL CANCER	111.5	116.3	124.2	121.8	153.6
BUC CAV & PHAR	1.9	1.8	1.9	1.8	2.6
ESOPHAGUS	1.8	2.0	2.8	1.3	3.2
STOMACH	32.6	21.4	23.6	15.3	16.1
COLON	6.4	6.0	6.2	10.2	10.9
RECTUM	2.6	2.3	3.8	3.5	4.1
LIVER & BIL	7.8	8.1	4.3	4.8	7.8
PANCREAS	6.4	9.2	9.7	12.5	12.0
LARYNX	1.7	1.8	1.2	1.6	1.4
TR, BR, & LUNG	10.1	14.5	18.2	20.1	28.8
OTHER RESPIR	0.3	0.3	0.9	0.3	0.1
BREAST	0.0	0.0	0.0	0.0	0.1
CERVIX	0.0	0.0	0.1	0.0	0.0
CORPUS UTERI	0.0	0.0	0.0	0.0	0.0
OTHER UTERUS	0.0	0.0	0.0	0.0	0.0
OVARY	0.0	0.0	0.0	0.0	0.0

(CONTINUED)

MORTALITY RATES

AVG ANNUAL AGE-ADJ (1970 US STANDARD) MORTALITY RATES/100,000
NEW MEXICO RESIDENTS, 1958-82, BY ETHNICITY, SEX, AND CAUSE

ETHNIC HISPANIC
AND SEX MALE

	YEAR_01				
	1958-62	1963-67	1968-72	1973-77	1978-82
	AGE_RATE	AGE_RATE	AGE_RATE	AGE_RATE	AGE_RATE
SITE	SUM	SUM	SUM	SUM	SUM
OTH FEM GEN	0.0	0.0	0.0	0.0	0.0
PROSTATE	11.4	14.1	17.3	14.3	19.8
TESTIS	0.8	0.8	1.1	0.2	0.4
OTH MALE GEN	0.5	0.3	0.8	0.1	0.2
KIDNEY	1.6	2.0	2.8	3.7	3.9
BLADDER	1.6	1.1	2.3	3.0	3.7
OTH URINARY	0.4	0.0	0.1	0.0	0.0
MELANOMA SKIN	0.3	0.3	0.6	0.3	0.2
OTHER SKIN	0.9	0.5	0.4	0.5	0.2
BRAIN	1.6	2.7	1.8	3.4	4.2
THYROID	0.5	0.8	0.3	0.3	0.4
BONE	1.3	1.9	1.3	0.7	0.5
LYMPH & RETIC	1.2	2.8	2.4	0.8	0.9
HODG LYMPH	1.1	1.2	1.9	1.4	1.3
LEUKEMIAS	4.0	6.9	3.9	4.9	5.9
OTH LYM & HEM	0.8	1.4	1.5	2.4	5.0
OTHER CANCER	10.6	11.0	11.5	13.2	18.7
OTH BRAIN CA	1.1	1.2	0.6	0.5	0.1
ALCOHOLISM	3.2	5.6	7.0	22.0	31.7
DIABETES	10.5	16.0	23.0	21.8	27.9

(CONTINUED)

APPENDIX

AVG ANNUAL AGE-ADJ (1970 US STANDARD) MORTALITY RATES/100,000
NEW MEXICO RESIDENTS, 1958-82, BY ETHNICITY, SEX, AND CAUSE

ETHNIC HISPANIC
AND SEX MALE

	YEAR_01				
	1958-62	1963-67	1968-72	1973-77	1978-82
	AGE_RATE	AGE_RATE	AGE_RATE	AGE_RATE	AGE_RATE
	SUM	SUM	SUM	SUM	SUM
SITE					
CIRCULATORY	327.3	356.7	390.1	326.4	280.0
RHEUM FEVER	0.2	0.1	0.1	0.6	0.4
CHRON RHM HRT	9.7	9.9	5.6	6.5	3.6
ISCHEMIC H D	143.8	167.4	220.7	187.1	144.0
HYPERTEN H D	17.9	17.8	7.5	2.7	4.9
HYPERTENSION	6.8	6.4	10.0	5.2	8.5
CEREBROVASC	82.9	75.8	82.5	65.5	48.9
OTH HRT & CIR	65.6	79.1	63.5	58.5	69.4
RESPIRATORY	77.4	73.8	88.1	88.5	76.6
ASTHMA	3.3	1.5	1.0	0.9	0.7
INFLUENZA	4.6	2.6	3.0	4.9	1.0
PNEUMONIA	50.9	44.7	56.9	52.2	34.0
CHR BRONCHI	0.9	1.1	1.1	0.4	0.1
EMPHYSEMA	4.0	10.3	10.8	7.1	5.6
COPD	0.0	0.0	1.0	12.9	24.3
OTH RESP DIS	13.4	13.4	14.0	9.8	10.6
PEPTIC ULCER	6.4	9.3	7.7	5.1	3.6
LIVER CIRRHO	19.6	26.2	45.1	40.2	31.8
NEPHRI -O	10.3	8.2	3.7	3.6	7.7
KIDNEY INFECT	4.3	5.0	4.5	1.5	0.9

(CONTINUED)

MORTALITY RATES

AVG ANNUAL AGE-ADJ (1970 US STANDARD) MORTALITY RATES/100,000
NEW MEXICO RESIDENTS, 1958-82, BY ETHNICITY, SEX, AND CAUSE

ETHNIC HISPANIC
AND SEX MALE

	YEAR_01				
	1958-62	1963-67	1968-72	1973-77	1978-82
	AGE_RATE	AGE_RATE	AGE_RATE	AGE_RATE	AGE_RATE
	SUM	SUM	SUM	SUM	SUM
SITE					
PREGNANCY CMP	0.0	0.0	0.0	0.0	0.0
CONGENITAL AN	12.2	9.6	10.1	6.9	6.7
DIS INFANCY	46.1	34.9	23.8	14.5	10.5
SYMP, ILL-DEF	95.3	80.8	52.3	56.9	58.3
OTH DIS, NEC	48.4	62.5	51.8	51.3	63.2
TL EXTERNAL	145.9	136.9	188.9	179.0	161.2
MOTOR VEH ACC	65.8	62.3	78.5	74.7	63.9
OTHER ACC	57.5	52.0	68.8	52.0	38.7
SUICIDE	10.7	10.9	18.2	24.2	25.4
HOMICIDE	11.5	10.4	20.2	23.0	27.5
LEGAL INTRVNT	0.2	1.0	0.8	0.0	0.5

AVG ANNUAL AGE-ADJ (1970 US STANDARD) MORTALITY RATES/100,000
NEW MEXICO RESIDENTS, 1958-82, BY ETHNICITY, SEX, AND CAUSE

ETHNIC HISPANIC
AND SEX FEMALE

	YEAR_01				
	1958-62	1963-67	1968-72	1973-77	1978-82
	AGE_RATE	AGE_RATE	AGE_RATE	AGE_RATE	AGE_RATE
	SUM	SUM	SUM	SUM	SUM
SITE					
ALL SITES	698.9	648.8	676.5	596.2	531.6
INF & PARA DIS	23.1	12.3	9.9	8.8	7.0
TUBERCULOSIS	10.3	4.3	2.2	2.3	1.1
INF & PARASIT	12.8	8.0	7.6	6.4	5.8
TOTAL CANCER	109.9	102.7	113.7	120.9	118.6
BUC CAV & PHAR	0.7	0.6	0.2	0.8	1.5
ESOPHAGUS	0.1	1.7	1.5	1.7	0.4
STOMACH	17.8	10.5	12.7	9.4	8.9
COLON	6.0	8.3	8.1	11.0	8.8
RECTUM	2.9	2.5	2.1	1.4	2.0
LIVER & BIL	12.8	9.8	8.7	9.3	8.2
PANCREAS	6.1	7.3	6.7	8.3	9.2
LARYNX	0.5	0.0	0.1	0.5	0.1
TR, BR, & LUNG	4.8	5.3	12.7	12.7	11.2
OTHER RESPIR	0.0	0.3	0.1	0.3	0.0
BREAST	10.2	11.9	13.3	14.4	19.4
CERVIX	10.6	9.8	8.1	7.6	4.4
CORPUS UTERI	0.8	0.9	0.9	0.9	1.5
OTHER UTERUS	3.7	2.4	3.6	1.9	1.0
OVARY	4.6	5.5	5.7	6.7	6.1

(CONTINUED)

MORTALITY RATES

AVG ANNUAL AGE-ADJ (1970 US STANDARD) MORTALITY RATES/100,000
NEW MEXICO RESIDENTS, 1958-82, BY ETHNICITY, SEX, AND CAUSE

ETHNIC HISPANIC
AND SEX FEMALE

	YEAR_01				
	1958-62	1963-67	1968-72	1973-77	1978-82
	AGE_RATE	AGE_RATE	AGE_RATE	AGE_RATE	AGE_RATE
SITE	SUM	SUM	SUM	SUM	SUM
OTH FEM GEN	2.0	0.7	0.1	0.5	0.8
PROSTATE	0.0	0.0	0.0	0.0	0.0
TESTIS	0.0	0.0	0.0	0.0	0.0
OTH MALE GEN	0.0	0.0	0.0	0.0	0.0
KIDNEY	1.0	1.3	1.7	2.0	1.6
BLADDER	1.8	1.5	0.8	1.5	1.3
OTH URINARY	0.0	0.3	0.0	0.1	0.2
MELANOMA SKIN	0.3	0.7	0.2	0.8	0.5
OTHER SKIN	0.2	0.5	0.7	0.4	0.4
BRAIN	0.7	2.0	1.8	2.1	1.8
THYROID	1.4	0.6	0.3	0.6	1.5
BONE	0.7	0.7	0.4	0.3	0.4
LYMPH & RETIC	2.3	1.2	1.5	1.3	1.1
HODG LYMPH	0.2	0.6	1.2	0.9	0.5
LEUKEMIAS	2.8	4.8	4.4	2.7	4.3
OTH LYM & HEM	1.1	0.9	2.8	2.1	3.5
OTHER CANCER	12.3	8.7	11.8	17.2	16.7
OTH BRAIN CA	1.1	0.8	1.7	1.4	0.6
ALCOHOLISM	0.5	0.8	0.9	2.9	4.6
DIABETES	15.7	19.8	27.3	24.5	28.6

(CONTINUED)

AVG ANNUAL AGE-ADJ (1970 US STANDARD) MORTALITY RATES/100,000
NEW MEXICO RESIDENTS, 1958-82, BY ETHNICITY, SEX, AND CAUSE

ETHNIC HISPANIC
AND SEX FEMALE

	YEAR_01				
	1958-62	1963-67	1968-72	1973-77	1978-82
	AGE_RATE	AGE_RATE	AGE_RATE	AGE_RATE	AGE_RATE
	SUM	SUM	SUM	SUM	SUM
SITE					
CIRCULATORY	275.0	262.5	289.1	232.8	186.8
RHEUM FEVER	0.4	0.3	0.4	0.4	1.0
CHRON RHM HRT	16.4	11.3	7.2	4.4	3.4
ISCHEMIC H D	91.4	107.8	136.0	104.9	82.3
HYPERTEN H D	21.9	20.2	6.5	1.6	4.7
HYPERTENSION	6.7	6.1	11.1	5.6	8.4
CEREBROVASC	74.6	62.7	76.5	66.9	43.8
OTH HRT & CIR	63.2	53.7	51.1	48.6	42.8
RESPIRATORY	57.9	53.6	64.5	56.0	41.0
ASTHMA	1.1	0.7	1.1	0.4	1.2
INFLUENZA	2.8	3.2	4.7	4.5	0.6
PNEUMONIA	38.4	32.6	39.9	33.8	21.0
CHR BRONCHI	0.6	1.5	1.3	0.2	0.0
EMPHYSEMA	2.2	4.6	6.5	3.7	2.3
COPD	0.0	0.0	0.3	8.7	11.3
OTH RESP DIS	12.6	10.8	10.4	4.3	4.3
PEPTIC ULCER	4.2	4.9	3.1	2.3	1.6
LIVER CIRRHO	8.5	9.2	12.6	7.7	11.1
NEPHRI -O	8.7	8.7	4.3	4.5	4.8
KIDNEY INFECT	2.7	5.8	3.8	0.9	0.3

(CONTINUED)

MORTALITY RATES

AVG ANNUAL AGE-ADJ (1970 US STANDARD) MORTALITY RATES/100,000
NEW MEXICO RESIDENTS, 1958-82, BY ETHNICITY, SEX, AND CAUSE

ETHNIC HISPANIC
AND SEX FEMALE

	1958-62 AGE_RATE SUM	1963-67 AGE_RATE SUM	1968-72 AGE_RATE SUM	1973-77 AGE_RATE SUM	1978-82 AGE_RATE SUM
SITE					
PREGNANCY CMP	1.5	0.5	0.7	0.8	0.6
CONGENITAL AN	8.8	8.7	7.0	6.6	4.9
DIS INFANCY	34.5	26.8	17.4	9.5	9.1
SYMP, ILL-DEF	64.9	40.9	27.9	31.1	30.9
OTH DIS, NEC	43.9	50.8	41.3	40.2	41.8
TL EXTERNAL	37.2	39.2	50.8	44.6	38.4
MOTOR VEH ACC	14.8	14.4	20.7	19.3	15.5
OTHER ACC	17.1	20.9	22.5	16.2	10.8
SUICIDE	1.8	1.4	3.7	4.0	5.9
HOMICIDE	3.4	2.3	3.3	4.2	4.7
LEGAL INTRVNT	0.0	0.0	0.0	0.0	0.0

(Columns under YEAR_01)

AVG ANNUAL AGE-ADJ (1970 US STANDARD) MORTALITY RATES/100,000
NEW MEXICO RESIDENTS, 1958-82, BY ETHNICITY, SEX, AND CAUSE

ETHNIC NONWHITE
AND SEX MALE

	YEAR_01				
	1958-62	1963-67	1968-72	1973-77	1978-82
	AGE_RATE	AGE_RATE	AGE_RATE	AGE_RATE	AGE_RATE
SITE	SUM	SUM	SUM	SUM	SUM
ALL SITES	1096.6	1078.5	1276.9	1355.0	1084.0
INF & PARA DIS	77.3	71.1	46.3	35.6	19.2
TUBERCULOSIS	38.0	31.5	23.3	18.4	7.1
INF & PARASIT	39.2	39.6	22.9	17.1	12.1
TOTAL CANCER	84.1	95.4	119.8	122.3	137.9
BUC CAV & PHAR	1.0	1.4	3.0	1.9	1.8
ESOPHAGUS	2.6	2.4	3.1	1.4	3.0
STOMACH	12.8	13.1	16.1	17.8	13.6
COLON	3.9	2.3	4.3	7.0	5.8
RECTUM	0.8	1.5	2.6	1.3	2.4
LIVER & BIL	6.8	8.9	6.7	6.2	14.7
PANCREAS	5.9	6.6	6.3	5.5	6.7
LARYNX	0.0	1.6	0.0	1.3	1.7
TR, BR, & LUNG	8.2	10.6	17.7	24.0	25.8
OTHER RESPIR	0.0	0.0	0.8	0.0	0.0
BREAST	1.0	0.0	0.0	0.0	0.6
CERVIX	0.0	0.0	0.0	0.0	0.0
CORPUS UTERI	0.0	0.0	0.0	0.0	0.0
OTHER UTERUS	0.0	0.0	0.0	0.0	0.0
OVARY	0.0	0.0	0.0	0.0	0.0

(CONTINUED)

MORTALITY RATES

AVG ANNUAL AGE-ADJ (1970 US STANDARD) MORTALITY RATES/100,000
NEW MEXICO RESIDENTS, 1958-82, BY ETHNICITY, SEX, AND CAUSE

ETHNIC NONWHITE
AND SEX MALE

SITE	1958-62 AGE_RATE SUM	1963-67 AGE_RATE SUM	1968-72 AGE_RATE SUM	1973-77 AGE_RATE SUM	1978-82 AGE_RATE SUM
OTH FEM GEN	0.0	0.0	0.0	0.0	0.0
PROSTATE	11.5	12.0	21.0	20.4	20.0
TESTIS	0.4	0.3	0.0	0.0	0.2
OTH MALE GEN	1.0	0.0	0.0	0.0	1.0
KIDNEY	6.0	4.8	4.6	5.1	2.4
BLADDER	0.8	1.6	2.4	1.3	0.6
OTH URINARY	0.0	0.0	0.7	0.0	0.0
MELANOMA SKIN	0.8	0.0	0.7	0.0	0.6
OTHER SKIN	1.0	0.0	0.7	0.0	0.0
BRAIN	1.4	0.3	3.6	1.2	3.4
THYROID	0.0	0.0	0.8	0.6	0.0
BONE	0.0	1.6	0.3	0.0	0.9
LYMPH & RETIC	2.1	3.7	3.1	2.0	0.6
HODG LYMPH	0.0	0.0	1.2	1.0	0.2
LEUKEMIAS	2.9	4.8	2.6	4.3	3.6
OTH LYM & HEM	0.8	1.5	2.9	4.3	5.3
OTHER CANCER	11.4	15.5	13.4	14.9	21.8
OTH BRAIN CA	0.3	2.5	1.0	0.0	0.0
ALCOHOLISM	10.3	7.9	25.4	81.8	66.5
DIABETES	13.2	10.9	25.8	22.5	24.2

(CONTINUED)

AVG ANNUAL AGE-ADJ (1970 US STANDARD) MORTALITY RATES/100,000 NEW MEXICO RESIDENTS, 1958-82, BY ETHNICITY, SEX, AND CAUSE

ETHNIC NONWHITE
AND SEX MALE

	YEAR_01				
	1958-62	1963-67	1968-72	1973-77	1978-82
	AGE_RATE	AGE_RATE	AGE_RATE	AGE_RATE	AGE_RATE
SITE	SUM	SUM	SUM	SUM	SUM
CIRCULATORY	260.5	237.0	299.7	286.2	225.5
RHEUM FEVER	1.3	0.7	0.0	1.6	0.2
CHRON RHM HRT	8.2	6.3	13.7	8.2	1.0
ISCHEMIC H D	103.3	89.3	124.1	124.1	94.9
HYPERTEN H D	16.8	10.7	3.2	3.7	3.1
HYPERTENSION	9.8	5.3	3.3	5.2	11.0
CEREBROVASC	69.3	67.2	94.9	70.7	40.8
OTH HRT & CIR	51.5	57.1	60.3	72.4	74.3
RESPIRATORY	96.4	77.6	112.2	113.2	77.8
ASTHMA	3.4	0.8	2.0	1.2	1.4
INFLUENZA	8.4	2.5	2.3	5.8	0.0
PNEUMONIA	68.0	55.2	76.7	74.3	38.3
CHR BRONCHI	1.0	1.5	1.5	2.1	0.0
EMPHYSEMA	0.0	5.2	3.7	2.8	2.9
COPD	0.0	0.0	1.5	11.0	11.2
OTH RESP DIS	15.3	12.1	24.1	15.6	23.9
PEPTIC ULCER	2.2	2.1	2.1	3.1	1.1
LIVER CIRRHO	13.8	18.0	55.7	63.7	27.4
NEPHRI -O	13.9	16.2	6.5	9.1	11.9
KIDNEY INFECT	11.3	8.6	4.8	2.1	1.7

(CONTINUED)

MORTALITY RATES

AVG ANNUAL AGE-ADJ (1970 US STANDARD) MORTALITY RATES/100,000
NEW MEXICO RESIDENTS, 1958-82, BY ETHNICITY, SEX, AND CAUSE

ETHNIC NONWHITE
AND SEX MALE

	YEAR_01				
	1958-62	1963-67	1968-72	1973-77	1978-82
	AGE_RATE	AGE_RATE	AGE_RATE	AGE_RATE	AGE_RATE
	SUM	SUM	SUM	SUM	SUM
SITE					
PREGNANCY CMP	0.0	0.0	0.0	0.0	0.0
CONGENITAL AN	9.4	13.0	9.8	7.6	9.2
DIS INFANCY	46.2	38.2	27.3	17.6	14.0
SYMP, ILL-DEF	151.9	154.9	112.1	119.0	99.0
OTH DIS, NEC	62.7	64.7	73.1	84.5	70.8
TL EXTERNAL	242.5	259.8	354.6	386.2	296.9
MOTOR VEH ACC	109.2	100.0	157.4	174.4	128.8
OTHER ACC	89.5	118.4	127.6	116.7	89.2
SUICIDE	18.1	15.7	26.0	37.3	30.2
HOMICIDE	25.6	24.6	38.3	45.8	39.9
LEGAL INTRVNT	0.0	0.9	0.6	0.5	0.4

AVG ANNUAL AGE-ADJ (1970 US STANDARD) MORTALITY RATES/100,000
NEW MEXICO RESIDENTS, 1958-82, BY ETHNICITY, SEX, AND CAUSE

ETHNIC NONWHITE
AND SEX FEMALE

	YEAR_01				
	1958-62	1963-67	1968-72	1973-77	1978-82
	AGE_RATE	AGE_RATE	AGE_RATE	AGE_RATE	AGE_RATE
SITE	SUM	SUM	SUM	SUM	SUM
ALL SITES	664.5	735.1	793.8	710.7	596.3
INF & PARA DIS	62.2	55.5	31.7	26.1	16.2
TUBERCULOSIS	29.7	23.0	12.7	9.2	7.1
INF & PARASIT	32.4	32.4	18.9	16.9	9.1
TOTAL CANCER	82.1	83.9	85.9	98.1	100.7
BUC CAV & PHAR	1.5	0.0	0.3	0.0	1.0
ESOPHAGUS	0.0	1.5	0.7	0.7	0.0
STOMACH	4.4	6.3	5.2	3.0	7.5
COLON	5.4	2.2	1.6	5.9	5.9
RECTUM	2.7	2.0	0.6	2.3	0.0
LIVER & BIL	13.8	11.6	10.6	14.5	12.5
PANCREAS	10.3	3.6	7.7	9.4	7.1
LARYNX	0.0	0.0	0.0	0.0	0.0
TR, BR, & LUNG	3.2	4.0	4.7	5.9	8.7
OTHER RESPIR	0.0	0.0	0.0	0.7	0.0
BREAST	8.2	9.0	14.7	11.3	11.3
CERVIX	5.1	9.8	7.0	5.1	6.7
CORPUS UTERI	1.2	0.0	0.7	0.0	1.4
OTHER UTERUS	3.2	4.4	0.7	0.0	0.5
OVARY	8.5	1.9	3.7	3.4	2.7

(CONTINUED)

AVG ANNUAL AGE-ADJ (1970 US STANDARD) MORTALITY RATES/100,000
NEW MEXICO RESIDENTS, 1958-82, BY ETHNICITY, SEX, AND CAUSE

ETHNIC NONWHITE
AND SEX FEMALE

	YEAR_01				
	1958-62	1963-67	1968-72	1973-77	1978-82
	AGE_RATE	AGE_RATE	AGE_RATE	AGE_RATE	AGE_RATE
SITE	SUM	SUM	SUM	SUM	SUM
OTH FEM GEN	0.0	0.0	1.5	1.6	1.7
PROSTATE	0.0	0.0	0.0	0.0	0.0
TESTIS	0.0	0.0	0.0	0.0	0.0
OTH MALE GEN	0.0	0.0	0.0	0.0	0.0
KIDNEY	0.8	1.9	0.7	2.0	2.1
BLADDER	0.9	1.5	0.5	0.5	0.0
OTH URINARY	0.0	0.0	0.0	0.7	0.0
MELANOMA SKIN	0.0	0.0	0.5	0.0	0.0
OTHER SKIN	0.0	0.0	0.0	0.0	0.8
BRAIN	0.0	0.2	0.0	1.0	0.2
THYROID	0.0	1.1	0.0	0.7	0.0
BONE	0.0	0.0	0.8	0.2	0.4
LYMPH & RETIC	0.0	1.1	0.7	0.0	0.0
HODG LYMPH	0.0	0.3	0.6	0.0	0.5
LEUKEMIAS	1.2	1.0	1.3	2.7	2.5
OTH LYM & HEM	1.2	1.9	3.0	4.2	4.0
OTHER CANCER	9.7	17.6	17.0	21.4	22.2
OTH BRAIN CA	1.5	0.3	1.7	0.9	0.6
ALCOHOLISM	2.5	2.0	6.3	21.3	16.0
DIABETES	6.6	12.4	27.6	22.5	29.7

(CONTINUED)

AVG ANNUAL AGE-ADJ (1970 US STANDARD) MORTALITY RATES/100,000
NEW MEXICO RESIDENTS, 1958-82, BY ETHNICITY, SEX, AND CAUSE

ETHNIC NONWHITE
AND SEX FEMALE

	YEAR_01				
	1958-62	1963-67	1968-72	1973-77	1978-82
	AGE_RATE	AGE_RATE	AGE_RATE	AGE_RATE	AGE_RATE
	SUM	SUM	SUM	SUM	SUM
SITE					
CIRCULATORY	149.7	173.1	241.4	183.1	135.6
RHEUM FEVER	1.4	0.3	0.6	0.7	0.5
CHRON RHM HRT	6.5	6.2	8.9	7.7	4.1
ISCHEMIC H D	46.9	59.6	95.7	65.9	44.1
HYPERTEN H D	14.2	17.7	3.1	0.0	3.0
HYPERTENSION	6.3	5.2	9.4	5.5	6.1
CEREBROVASC	50.1	38.3	71.6	53.8	35.5
OTH HRT & CIR	24.0	45.4	51.8	49.2	41.9
RESPIRATORY	69.4	57.6	75.5	55.8	43.5
ASTHMA	0.0	0.7	0.6	0.5	1.6
INFLUENZA	5.0	1.2	1.9	2.2	0.4
PNEUMONIA	53.6	46.1	49.5	39.1	27.7
CHR BRONCHI	1.2	0.7	0.2	0.7	0.0
EMPHYSEMA	0.0	1.5	0.5	0.6	0.0
COPD	0.0	0.0	1.6	4.7	4.0
OTH RESP DIS	9.4	7.1	21.0	7.8	9.7
PEPTIC ULCER	1.8	2.9	0.6	2.9	2.3
LIVER CIRRHO	9.5	19.0	34.8	30.7	14.1
NEPHRI -O	9.3	13.9	10.7	7.0	14.3
KIDNEY INFECT	9.3	11.4	7.5	2.8	0.6

(CONTINUED)

MORTALITY RATES

AVG ANNUAL AGE-ADJ (1970 US STANDARD) MORTALITY RATES/100,000
NEW MEXICO RESIDENTS, 1958-82, BY ETHNICITY, SEX, AND CAUSE

ETHNIC NONWHITE
AND SEX FEMALE

	YEAR_01				
	1958-62	1963-67	1968-72	1973-77	1978-82
	AGE_RATE SUM	AGE_RATE SUM	AGE_RATE SUM	AGE_RATE SUM	AGE_RATE SUM
SITE					
PREGNANCY CMP	1.6	1.7	2.8	0.5	1.4
CONGENITAL AN	7.9	6.9	5.7	7.8	5.6
DIS INFANCY	36.5	29.3	21.0	12.3	7.2
SYMP, ILL-DEF	93.6	119.6	76.7	67.8	68.9
OTH DIS, NEC	54.8	58.4	53.7	70.4	57.0
TL EXTERNAL	65.4	86.4	109.5	99.9	81.9
MOTOR VEH ACC	27.6	36.4	55.4	51.9	45.5
OTHER ACC	26.1	38.0	36.9	26.1	24.2
SUICIDE	2.9	2.3	4.0	5.2	2.7
HOMICIDE	8.7	9.5	11.3	12.8	6.4
LEGAL INTRVNT	0.0	0.0	0.5	0.0	0.0

AVG ANNUAL AGE-ADJ (1970 US STANDARD) MORTALITY RATES/100,000
NEW MEXICO RESIDENTS, 1958-82, BY ETHNICITY, SEX, AND CAUSE

ETHNIC INDIAN
AND SEX MALE

	YEAR_01				
	1958-62	1963-67	1968-72	1973-77	1978-82
	AGE_RATE	AGE_RATE	AGE_RATE	AGE_RATE	AGE_RATE
	SUM	SUM	SUM	SUM	SUM
SITE					
ALL SITES	1098.9	1111.9	1332.9	1494.5	1153.2
INF & PARA DIS	88.8	90.8	56.1	44.2	21.8
TUBERCULOSIS	45.7	42.5	27.6	23.5	8.5
INF & PARASIT	43.0	48.2	28.4	20.7	13.2
TOTAL CANCER	81.7	82.9	92.8	96.3	112.2
BUC CAV & PHAR	0.0	0.0	2.2	1.2	0.0
ESOPHAGUS	2.4	0.0	0.0	1.8	2.4
STOMACH	12.8	13.9	16.0	17.5	16.1
COLON	2.6	2.1	1.5	5.7	4.4
RECTUM	0.0	1.0	2.7	0.9	1.6
LIVER & BIL	9.2	12.1	8.7	5.5	18.9
PANCREAS	2.7	5.6	3.1	2.9	4.8
LARYNX	0.0	0.0	0.0	0.0	0.8
TR, BR, & LUNG	5.3	4.7	9.0	7.7	10.8
OTHER RESPIR	0.0	0.0	1.1	0.0	0.0
BREAST	0.0	0.0	0.0	0.0	0.0
CERVIX	0.0	0.0	0.0	0.0	0.0
CORPUS UTERI	0.0	0.0	0.0	0.0	0.0
OTHER UTERUS	0.0	0.0	0.0	0.0	0.0
OVARY	0.0	0.0	0.0	0.0	0.0

(CONTINUED)

MORTALITY RATES

AVG ANNUAL AGE-ADJ (1970 US STANDARD) MORTALITY RATES/100,000
NEW MEXICO RESIDENTS, 1958-82, BY ETHNICITY, SEX, AND CAUSE

ETHNIC INDIAN
AND SEX MALE

	\multicolumn{5}{c}{YEAR_01}
	1958-62	1963-67	1968-72	1973-77	1978-82
	AGE_RATE SUM	AGE_RATE SUM	AGE_RATE SUM	AGE_RATE SUM	AGE_RATE SUM
SITE					
OTH FEM GEN	0.0	0.0	0.0	0.0	0.0
PROSTATE	12.3	7.6	11.0	17.4	15.2
TESTIS	0.6	0.4	0.0	0.0	0.3
OTH MALE GEN	1.3	0.0	0.0	0.0	1.4
KIDNEY	6.4	5.3	5.3	6.0	2.5
BLADDER	1.2	0.0	1.1	0.9	0.0
OTH URINARY	0.0	0.0	1.0	0.0	0.0
MELANOMA SKIN	1.2	0.0	1.0	0.0	0.8
OTHER SKIN	1.3	0.0	1.0	0.0	0.0
BRAIN	1.7	0.4	3.2	1.7	1.5
THYROID	0.0	0.0	1.1	0.9	0.0
BONE	0.0	2.2	0.4	0.0	1.1
LYMPH & RETIC	2.5	4.0	2.0	1.8	0.0
HODG LYMPH	0.0	0.0	0.0	0.9	0.0
LEUKEMIAS	3.4	5.2	2.5	3.9	2.6
OTH LYM & HEM	0.0	0.0	4.0	3.1	3.6
OTHER CANCER	14.0	17.8	14.0	15.5	22.5
OTH BRAIN CA	0.3	3.5	0.4	0.0	0.0
ALCOHOLISM	9.7	11.1	30.6	108.1	77.6
DIABETES	11.6	10.5	26.2	24.9	22.4

(CONTINUED)

AVG ANNUAL AGE-ADJ (1970 US STANDARD) MORTALITY RATES/100,000
NEW MEXICO RESIDENTS, 1958-82, BY ETHNICITY, SEX, AND CAUSE

ETHNIC INDIAN
AND SEX MALE

	YEAR_01				
	1958-62	1963-67	1968-72	1973-77	1978-82
	AGE_RATE	AGE_RATE	AGE_RATE	AGE_RATE	AGE_RATE
SITE	SUM	SUM	SUM	SUM	SUM
CIRCULATORY	201.7	186.3	243.0	247.1	198.7
RHEUM FEVER	0.6	1.0	0.0	1.3	0.2
CHRON RHM HRT	10.2	6.3	14.9	10.0	1.4
ISCHEMIC H D	85.5	62.8	100.5	98.4	68.3
HYPERTEN H D	8.0	7.6	0.0	1.9	1.6
HYPERTENSION	3.2	1.1	3.3	4.1	8.1
CEREBROVASC	52.2	54.2	70.1	58.8	39.8
OTH HRT & CIR	41.7	53.0	54.0	72.3	79.0
RESPIRATORY	110.2	89.7	112.3	126.9	87.0
ASTHMA	1.1	0.0	0.7	0.0	1.6
INFLUENZA	8.4	2.2	0.9	5.8	0.0
PNEUMONIA	80.9	64.9	81.2	89.3	45.0
CHR BRONCHI	1.3	2.1	1.1	1.9	0.0
EMPHYSEMA	0.0	5.9	0.9	0.0	2.1
COPD	0.0	0.0	2.0	11.9	10.0
OTH RESP DIS	18.1	14.5	25.0	17.7	28.1
PEPTIC ULCER	1.9	0.0	0.9	2.3	1.6
LIVER CIRRHO	14.2	18.6	69.7	86.5	35.8
NEPHRI -O	10.7	18.4	9.0	9.3	14.4
KIDNEY INFECT	10.2	8.3	4.4	0.9	2.5

(CONTINUED)

AVG ANNUAL AGE-ADJ (1970 US STANDARD) MORTALITY RATES/100,000
NEW MEXICO RESIDENTS, 1958-82, BY ETHNICITY, SEX, AND CAUSE

ETHNIC INDIAN
AND SEX MALE

	YEAR_01				
	1958-62	1963-67	1968-72	1973-77	1978-82
	AGE_RATE	AGE_RATE	AGE_RATE	AGE_RATE	AGE_RATE
	SUM	SUM	SUM	SUM	SUM
SITE					
PREGNANCY CMP	0.0	0.0	0.0	0.0	0.0
CONGENITAL AN	10.3	13.9	9.5	8.7	9.7
DIS INFANCY	43.1	35.1	24.8	13.1	13.3
SYMP, ILL-DEF	155.1	173.3	129.5	139.4	115.6
OTH DIS, NEC	68.9	69.5	84.8	97.0	76.3
TL EXTERNAL	279.6	299.5	438.2	488.9	363.7
MOTOR VEH ACC	128.8	122.3	203.4	233.0	166.9
OTHER ACC	108.4	143.7	164.8	143.8	109.4
SUICIDE	25.0	18.7	33.1	48.8	35.7
HOMICIDE	17.2	14.1	29.9	46.5	39.7
LEGAL INTRVNT	0.0	0.4	0.4	0.7	0.5

AVG ANNUAL AGE-ADJ (1970 US STANDARD) MORTALITY RATES/100,000
NEW MEXICO RESIDENTS, 1958-82, BY ETHNICITY, SEX, AND CAUSE

ETHNIC INDIAN
AND SEX FEMALE

	YEAR_01				
	1958-62	1963-67	1968-72	1973-77	1978-82
	AGE_RATE	AGE_RATE	AGE_RATE	AGE_RATE	AGE_RATE
	SUM	SUM	SUM	SUM	SUM
SITE					
ALL SITES	671.4	759.8	798.1	742.3	622.6
INF & PARA DIS	80.0	73.1	38.8	33.6	20.0
TUBERCULOSIS	40.0	31.6	16.0	12.7	9.6
INF & PARASIT	40.0	41.4	22.8	20.8	10.3
TOTAL CANCER	68.4	82.1	81.3	94.5	92.6
BUC CAV & PHAR	0.0	0.0	0.4	0.0	0.0
ESOPHAGUS	0.0	2.2	0.0	0.0	0.0
STOMACH	6.1	5.8	3.1	4.1	9.4
COLON	3.1	2.2	0.0	2.9	4.6
RECTUM	0.0	1.6	0.0	2.4	0.0
LIVER & BIL	18.6	16.1	13.6	19.2	15.5
PANCREAS	6.8	2.1	6.6	10.1	7.3
LARYNX	0.0	0.0	0.0	0.0	0.0
TR, BR, & LUNG	1.6	1.9	5.6	2.3	4.2
OTHER RESPIR	0.0	0.0	0.0	0.9	0.0
BREAST	2.5	4.4	12.6	8.8	8.9
CERVIX	3.8	9.8	7.8	5.9	7.7
CORPUS UTERI	1.6	0.0	0.0	0.0	0.6
OTHER UTERUS	1.6	2.2	0.0	0.0	0.0
OVARY	8.6	1.4	2.1	2.7	2.1

(CONTINUED)

MORTALITY RATES

AVG ANNUAL AGE-ADJ (1970 US STANDARD) MORTALITY RATES/100,000
NEW MEXICO RESIDENTS, 1958-82, BY ETHNICITY, SEX, AND CAUSE

ETHNIC INDIAN
AND SEX FEMALE

	YEAR_01				
	1958-62	1963-67	1968-72	1973-77	1978-82
	AGE_RATE	AGE_RATE	AGE_RATE	AGE_RATE	AGE_RATE
SITE	SUM	SUM	SUM	SUM	SUM
OTH FEM GEN	0.0	0.0	2.1	0.6	1.5
PROSTATE	0.0	0.0	0.0	0.0	0.0
TESTIS	0.0	0.0	0.0	0.0	0.0
OTH MALE GEN	0.0	0.0	0.0	0.0	0.0
KIDNEY	1.2	2.7	0.0	2.7	2.8
BLADDER	0.0	2.0	0.0	0.7	0.0
OTH URINARY	0.0	0.0	0.0	0.0	0.0
MELANOMA SKIN	0.0	0.0	0.8	0.0	0.0
OTHER SKIN	0.0	0.0	0.0	0.0	0.3
BRAIN	0.0	0.3	0.0	0.3	0.2
THYROID	0.0	0.9	0.0	1.0	0.0
BONE	0.0	0.0	1.1	0.3	0.5
LYMPH & RETIC	0.0	1.5	1.0	0.0	0.0
HODG LYMPH	0.0	0.0	0.0	0.0	0.0
LEUKEMIAS	1.2	0.9	1.8	3.3	1.7
OTH LYM & HEM	0.0	0.9	3.0	4.1	3.9
OTHER CANCER	10.9	22.5	19.1	21.4	20.4
OTH BRAIN CA	2.2	0.4	0.0	1.2	0.8
ALCOHOLISM	2.4	1.9	8.8	29.7	19.9
DIABETES	6.6	7.7	26.0	18.0	32.2

(CONTINUED)

AVG ANNUAL AGE-ADJ (1970 US STANDARD) MORTALITY RATES/100,000
NEW MEXICO RESIDENTS, 1958-82, BY ETHNICITY, SEX, AND CAUSE

ETHNIC INDIAN
AND SEX FEMALE

	YEAR_01				
	1958-62	1963-67	1968-72	1973-77	1978-82
	AGE_RATE	AGE_RATE	AGE_RATE	AGE_RATE	AGE_RATE
	SUM	SUM	SUM	SUM	SUM
SITE					
CIRCULATORY	109.6	138.7	178.5	147.5	114.8
RHEUM FEVER	1.9	0.4	0.9	0.0	0.7
CHRON RHM HRT	6.6	7.8	10.6	8.5	4.7
ISCHEMIC H D	37.6	40.0	57.1	39.4	26.5
HYPERTEN H D	8.9	11.2	2.4	0.0	0.5
HYPERTENSION	2.6	2.1	5.4	2.4	3.7
CEREBROVASC	36.5	32.8	55.7	43.9	34.6
OTH HRT & CIR	15.2	44.0	46.1	53.2	43.8
RESPIRATORY	84.9	65.3	89.7	67.4	49.6
ASTHMA	0.0	0.0	0.0	0.0	0.8
INFLUENZA	5.0	1.6	2.5	3.0	0.6
PNEUMONIA	66.1	55.3	61.8	47.1	34.6
CHR BRONCHI	1.6	1.0	0.3	0.9	0.0
EMPHYSEMA	0.0	1.2	0.0	0.0	0.0
COPD	0.0	0.0	0.0	5.7	0.8
OTH RESP DIS	12.0	6.1	25.0	10.5	12.6
PEPTIC ULCER	2.5	4.1	0.9	1.8	1.5
LIVER CIRRHO	12.6	20.7	41.4	38.6	17.7
NEPHRI -O	8.6	13.3	9.4	7.1	16.2
KIDNEY INFECT	12.2	14.9	7.6	3.9	0.0

(CONTINUED)

MORTALITY RATES

AVG ANNUAL AGE-ADJ (1970 US STANDARD) MORTALITY RATES/100,000
NEW MEXICO RESIDENTS, 1958-82, BY ETHNICITY, SEX, AND CAUSE

ETHNIC INDIAN
AND SEX FEMALE

	YEAR_01				
	1958-62	1963-67	1968-72	1973-77	1978-82
	AGE_RATE	AGE_RATE	AGE_RATE	AGE_RATE	AGE_RATE
	SUM	SUM	SUM	SUM	SUM
SITE					
PREGNANCY CMP	1.7	2.4	3.0	0.3	1.2
CONGENITAL AN	8.0	6.4	6.6	7.3	6.2
DIS INFANCY	33.2	27.9	22.2	10.8	7.0
SYMP, ILL-DEF	105.0	138.1	93.4	80.4	81.7
OTH DIS, NEC	62.6	60.7	64.5	79.8	62.6
TL EXTERNAL	70.2	101.5	125.3	119.7	97.8
MOTOR VEH ACC	32.1	47.8	67.1	65.5	56.9
OTHER ACC	31.0	45.2	42.1	30.5	29.0
SUICIDE	1.0	1.6	3.1	6.1	2.7
HOMICIDE	5.9	6.7	12.3	12.5	5.3
LEGAL INTRVNT	0.0	0.0	0.0	0.0	0.0

AVG ANNUAL AGE-ADJ (1970 US STANDARD) MORTALITY RATES/100,000
NEW MEXICO RESIDENTS, 1958-82, BY ETHNICITY, SEX, AND CAUSE

ETHNIC BLACK
AND SEX MALE

	YEAR_01				
	1958-62	1963-67	1968-72	1973-77	1978-82
	AGE_RATE	AGE_RATE	AGE_RATE	AGE_RATE	AGE_RATE
SITE	SUM	SUM	SUM	SUM	SUM
ALL SITES	1281.1	1173.1	1384.8	1209.6	1028.9
INF & PARA DIS	49.7	15.0	17.0	12.4	13.1
TUBERCULOSIS	17.3	0.0	9.2	4.1	3.4
INF & PARASIT	32.3	15.0	7.7	8.2	9.7
TOTAL CANCER	114.0	156.1	240.3	233.9	238.3
BUC CAV & PHAR	0.0	6.6	5.9	4.5	5.3
ESOPHAGUS	3.4	10.7	12.7	0.0	5.5
STOMACH	15.1	14.1	21.5	25.8	5.2
COLON	9.9	3.6	11.5	12.8	12.3
RECTUM	3.4	3.4	3.1	2.7	6.2
LIVER & BIL	0.0	0.0	0.0	9.2	0.0
PANCREAS	20.7	10.9	18.7	15.2	15.0
LARYNX	0.0	7.4	0.0	6.3	5.3
TR, BR, & LUNG	23.0	30.4	52.8	83.8	78.9
OTHER RESPIR	0.0	0.0	0.0	0.0	0.0
BREAST	6.3	0.0	0.0	0.0	3.4
CERVIX	0.0	0.0	0.0	0.0	0.0
CORPUS UTERI	0.0	0.0	0.0	0.0	0.0
OTHER UTERUS	0.0	0.0	0.0	0.0	0.0
OVARY	0.0	0.0	0.0	0.0	0.0

(CONTINUED)

MORTALITY RATES

AVG ANNUAL AGE-ADJ (1970 US STANDARD) MORTALITY RATES/100,000
NEW MEXICO RESIDENTS, 1958-82, BY ETHNICITY, SEX, AND CAUSE

ETHNIC BLACK
AND SEX MALE

	YEAR_01				
	1958-62	1963-67	1968-72	1973-77	1978-82
	AGE_RATE	AGE_RATE	AGE_RATE	AGE_RATE	AGE_RATE
	SUM	SUM	SUM	SUM	SUM
SITE					
OTH FEM GEN	0.0	0.0	0.0	0.0	0.0
PROSTATE	12.7	30.3	63.4	36.8	42.0
TESTIS	0.0	0.0	0.0	0.0	0.0
OTH MALE GEN	0.0	0.0	0.0	0.0	0.0
KIDNEY	6.3	3.4	2.9	0.0	3.4
BLADDER	0.0	8.4	7.9	3.1	3.4
OTH URINARY	0.0	0.0	0.0	0.0	0.0
MELANOMA SKIN	0.0	0.0	0.0	0.0	0.0
OTHER SKIN	0.0	0.0	0.0	0.0	0.0
BRAIN	1.4	0.0	6.2	0.0	9.6
THYROID	0.0	0.0	0.0	0.0	0.0
BONE	0.0	0.0	0.0	0.0	0.0
LYMPH & RETIC	1.4	3.4	8.6	3.1	2.7
HODG LYMPH	0.0	0.0	5.3	1.3	1.1
LEUKEMIAS	1.8	4.8	3.4	6.2	7.4
OTH LYM & HEM	3.4	6.7	0.0	6.9	9.6
OTHER CANCER	4.4	11.1	15.7	15.3	20.9
OTH BRAIN CA	0.0	0.0	0.0	0.0	0.0
ALCOHOLISM	14.2	0.0	16.6	17.2	48.9
DIABETES	22.0	7.8	31.4	21.6	36.4

(CONTINUED)

AVG ANNUAL AGE-ADJ (1970 US STANDARD) MORTALITY RATES/100,000
NEW MEXICO RESIDENTS, 1958-82, BY ETHNICITY, SEX, AND CAUSE

ETHNIC BLACK
AND SEX MALE

	YEAR_01				
	1958-62	1963-67	1968-72	1973-77	1978-82
	AGE_RATE	AGE_RATE	AGE_RATE	AGE_RATE	AGE_RATE
	SUM	SUM	SUM	SUM	SUM
SITE					
CIRCULATORY	478.3	441.2	539.9	463.2	341.7
RHEUM FEVER	3.3	0.0	0.0	3.0	0.0
CHRON RHM HRT	3.4	8.0	13.7	4.0	0.0
ISCHEMIC H D	164.2	190.0	233.1	231.6	188.1
HYPERTEN H D	46.4	22.8	8.3	11.5	6.2
HYPERTENSION	36.3	21.0	3.5	12.5	22.0
CEREBROVASC	128.2	113.8	196.0	117.8	51.4
OTH HRT & CIR	96.4	85.3	85.1	82.4	73.9
RESPIRATORY	55.9	46.1	120.3	81.3	53.6
ASTHMA	10.8	4.2	6.6	5.9	1.2
INFLUENZA	4.4	3.8	7.2	7.3	0.0
PNEUMONIA	33.1	27.4	64.9	33.2	20.6
CHR BRONCHI	0.0	0.0	3.1	3.1	0.0
EMPHYSEMA	0.0	3.6	11.2	10.2	6.2
COPD	0.0	0.0	0.0	9.4	14.5
OTH RESP DIS	7.5	6.8	27.2	11.9	10.9
PEPTIC ULCER	3.4	6.5	6.3	6.3	0.0
LIVER CIRRHO	17.0	13.1	29.9	8.9	6.8
NEPHRI -O	28.5	13.0	0.0	11.7	4.9
KIDNEY INFECT	17.9	11.4	7.3	6.4	0.0

(CONTINUED)

MORTALITY RATES

AVG ANNUAL AGE-ADJ (1970 US STANDARD) MORTALITY RATES/100,000
NEW MEXICO RESIDENTS, 1958-82, BY ETHNICITY, SEX, AND CAUSE

ETHNIC BLACK
AND SEX MALE

SITE	YEAR_01				
	1958-62	1963-67	1968-72	1973-77	1978-82
	AGE_RATE	AGE_RATE	AGE_RATE	AGE_RATE	AGE_RATE
	SUM	SUM	SUM	SUM	SUM
PREGNANCY CMP	0.0	0.0	0.0	0.0	0.0
CONGENITAL AN	5.6	14.4	14.0	5.4	8.7
DIS INFANCY	70.6	65.0	42.8	42.5	22.5
SYMP, ILL-DEF	159.6	119.8	81.7	77.7	56.6
OTH DIS, NEC	50.0	60.3	48.4	64.8	56.1
TL EXTERNAL	193.5	202.7	188.1	155.6	140.6
MOTOR VEH ACC	78.2	54.5	58.1	31.6	30.4
OTHER ACC	53.1	67.4	38.4	54.7	43.7
SUICIDE	4.4	11.8	11.3	9.8	15.4
HOMICIDE	57.7	65.7	78.8	59.4	51.0
LEGAL INTRVNT	0.0	3.2	1.3	0.0	0.0

AVG ANNUAL AGE-ADJ (1970 US STANDARD) MORTALITY RATES/100,000
NEW MEXICO RESIDENTS, 1958-82, BY ETHNICITY, SEX, AND CAUSE

ETHNIC BLACK
AND SEX FEMALE

	YEAR_01				
	1958-62	1963-67	1968-72	1973-77	1978-82
	AGE_RATE	AGE_RATE	AGE_RATE	AGE_RATE	AGE_RATE
SITE	SUM	SUM	SUM	SUM	SUM
ALL SITES	783.7	844.7	965.7	764.3	598.5
INF & PARA DIS	16.6	6.8	13.3	5.7	4.1
TUBERCULOSIS	3.3	0.0	3.0	0.0	0.0
INF & PARASIT	13.2	6.8	10.3	5.7	4.1
TOTAL CANCER	141.5	115.6	121.0	129.6	138.9
BUC CAV & PHAR	6.6	0.0	0.0	0.0	1.9
ESOPHAGUS	0.0	0.0	3.4	3.4	0.0
STOMACH	0.0	9.0	13.3	0.0	2.7
COLON	14.3	3.0	7.3	12.2	11.3
RECTUM	12.4	4.0	3.0	2.5	0.0
LIVER & BIL	1.9	0.0	3.4	3.4	2.8
PANCREAS	23.5	9.6	13.3	9.4	8.3
LARYNX	0.0	0.0	0.0	0.0	0.0
TR, BR, & LUNG	8.5	11.9	3.0	19.2	25.7
OTHER RESPIR	0.0	0.0	0.0	0.0	0.0
BREAST	25.7	27.5	26.3	22.9	22.7
CERVIX	10.1	11.4	7.5	2.6	4.7
CORPUS UTERI	0.0	0.0	3.4	0.0	3.8
OTHER UTERUS	8.1	13.7	2.9	0.0	2.5
OVARY	10.6	5.3	7.0	6.9	5.3

(CONTINUED)

MORTALITY RATES

AVG ANNUAL AGE-ADJ (1970 US STANDARD) MORTALITY RATES/100,000
NEW MEXICO RESIDENTS, 1958-82, BY ETHNICITY, SEX, AND CAUSE

ETHNIC BLACK
AND SEX FEMALE

	YEAR_01				
	1958-62	1963-67	1968-72	1973-77	1978-82
	AGE_RATE	AGE_RATE	AGE_RATE	AGE_RATE	AGE_RATE
SITE	SUM	SUM	SUM	SUM	SUM
OTH FEM GEN	0.0	0.0	0.0	5.3	2.8
PROSTATE	0.0	0.0	0.0	0.0	0.0
TESTIS	0.0	0.0	0.0	0.0	0.0
OTH MALE GEN	0.0	0.0	0.0	0.0	0.0
KIDNEY	0.0	0.0	3.4	0.0	0.0
BLADDER	4.0	0.0	3.0	0.0	0.0
OTH URINARY	0.0	0.0	0.0	3.4	0.0
MELANOMA SKIN	0.0	0.0	0.0	0.0	0.0
OTHER SKIN	0.0	0.0	0.0	0.0	2.5
BRAIN	0.0	0.0	0.0	3.4	0.0
THYROID	0.0	2.6	0.0	0.0	0.0
BONE	0.0	0.0	0.0	0.0	0.0
LYMPH & RETIC	0.0	0.0	0.0	0.0	0.0
HODG LYMPH	0.0	2.1	3.0	0.0	0.0
LEUKEMIAS	2.0	2.1	0.0	1.8	5.6
OTH LYM & HEM	5.8	6.2	3.9	6.0	4.7
OTHER CANCER	7.3	6.7	13.3	26.6	30.8
OTH BRAIN CA	0.0	0.0	8.3	0.0	0.0
ALCOHOLISM	3.3	3.0	0.0	0.0	8.3
DIABETES	8.5	31.1	40.8	40.3	27.9

(CONTINUED)

AVG ANNUAL AGE-ADJ (1970 US STANDARD) MORTALITY RATES/100,000
NEW MEXICO RESIDENTS, 1958-82, BY ETHNICITY, SEX, AND CAUSE

ETHNIC BLACK
AND SEX FEMALE

	YEAR_01				
	1958-62	1963-67	1968-72	1973-77	1978-82
	AGE_RATE	AGE_RATE	AGE_RATE	AGE_RATE	AGE_RATE
	SUM	SUM	SUM	SUM	SUM
SITE					
CIRCULATORY	315.8	328.9	496.6	334.5	216.8
RHEUM FEVER	0.0	0.0	0.0	3.4	0.0
CHRON RHM HRT	8.0	3.4	6.4	6.0	2.8
ISCHEMIC H D	86.7	130.9	237.8	164.7	100.8
HYPERTEN H D	36.2	43.5	6.4	0.0	12.0
HYPERTENSION	19.9	17.8	24.8	18.0	16.8
CEREBROVASC	105.7	68.6	135.8	93.5	42.4
OTH HRT & CIR	59.1	64.5	85.2	48.6	41.8
RESPIRATORY	30.3	46.5	48.7	30.5	26.6
ASTHMA	0.0	4.5	3.0	2.6	5.1
INFLUENZA	6.5	0.0	0.0	0.0	0.0
PNEUMONIA	21.1	25.5	21.2	21.2	6.9
CHR BRONCHI	0.0	0.0	0.0	0.0	0.0
EMPHYSEMA	0.0	2.9	3.0	2.5	0.0
COPD	0.0	0.0	7.3	2.7	12.6
OTH RESP DIS	2.7	13.6	14.0	1.4	1.8
PEPTIC ULCER	0.0	0.0	0.0	8.0	5.5
LIVER CIRRHO	3.3	19.4	25.5	15.2	6.6
NEPHRI -O	13.4	17.7	15.0	8.7	12.2
KIDNEY INFECT	2.1	3.9	9.9	0.0	2.8

(CONTINUED)

MORTALITY RATES

AVG ANNUAL AGE-ADJ (1970 US STANDARD) MORTALITY RATES/100,000
NEW MEXICO RESIDENTS, 1958-82, BY ETHNICITY, SEX, AND CAUSE

ETHNIC BLACK
AND SEX FEMALE

	YEAR_01				
	1958-62	1963-67	1968-72	1973-77	1978-82
	AGE_RATE	AGE_RATE	AGE_RATE	AGE_RATE	AGE_RATE
	SUM	SUM	SUM	SUM	SUM
SITE					
PREGNANCY CMP	2.2	0.0	1.9	1.5	3.0
CONGENITAL AN	9.5	10.1	1.5	10.0	4.0
DIS INFANCY	55.6	39.2	20.2	24.0	10.8
SYMP, ILL-DEF	74.2	89.5	42.0	43.7	37.1
OTH DIS, NEC	42.4	67.2	30.6	57.0	54.1
TL EXTERNAL	64.4	65.0	89.5	54.8	39.2
MOTOR VEH ACC	18.2	8.3	31.4	13.6	13.8
OTHER ACC	16.7	24.2	28.9	18.1	12.5
SUICIDE	6.8	6.5	9.1	1.6	1.2
HOMICIDE	22.6	25.9	11.7	19.8	11.5
LEGAL INTRVNT	0.0	0.0	3.0	0.0	0.0

AVG ANNUAL AGE-ADJ (1970 US STANDARD) MORTALITY RATES/100,000
NEW MEXICO RESIDENTS, 1958-82, BY ETHNICITY, SEX, AND CAUSE

ETHNIC OTH NW
AND SEX MALE

	YEAR_01				
	1958-62	1963-67	1968-72	1973-77	1978-82
	AGE_RATE	AGE_RATE	AGE_RATE	AGE_RATE	AGE_RATE
	SUM	SUM	SUM	SUM	SUM
SITE					
ALL SITES	398.0	288.3	325.3	294.5	353.6
INF & PARA DIS	17.5	0.0	12.7	0.0	3.9
TUBERCULOSIS	17.5	0.0	12.7	0.0	0.0
INF & PARASIT	0.0	0.0	0.0	0.0	3.9
TOTAL CANCER	21.7	6.8	29.1	25.0	91.1
BUC CAV & PHAR	21.7	0.0	0.0	0.0	16.1
ESOPHAGUS	0.0	0.0	12.7	0.0	0.0
STOMACH	0.0	0.0	0.0	0.0	15.5
COLON	0.0	0.0	16.4	0.0	0.0
RECTUM	0.0	0.0	0.0	0.0	0.0
LIVER & BIL	0.0	0.0	0.0	0.0	15.5
PANCREAS	0.0	0.0	0.0	0.0	0.0
LARYNX	0.0	0.0	0.0	0.0	0.0
TR, BR, & LUNG	0.0	6.8	0.0	0.0	11.3
OTHER RESPIR	0.0	0.0	0.0	0.0	0.0
BREAST	0.0	0.0	0.0	0.0	0.0
CERVIX	0.0	0.0	0.0	0.0	0.0
CORPUS UTERI	0.0	0.0	0.0	0.0	0.0
OTHER UTERUS	0.0	0.0	0.0	0.0	0.0
OVARY	0.0	0.0	0.0	0.0	0.0

(CONTINUED)

MORTALITY RATES

AVG ANNUAL AGE-ADJ (1970 US STANDARD) MORTALITY RATES/100,000
NEW MEXICO RESIDENTS, 1958-82, BY ETHNICITY, SEX, AND CAUSE

ETHNIC OTH NW
AND SEX MALE

	YEAR_01				
	1958-62	1963-67	1968-72	1973-77	1978-82
	AGE_RATE	AGE_RATE	AGE_RATE	AGE_RATE	AGE_RATE
	SUM	SUM	SUM	SUM	SUM
SITE					
OTH FEM GEN	0.0	0.0	0.0	0.0	0.0
PROSTATE	0.0	0.0	0.0	0.0	0.0
TESTIS	0.0	0.0	0.0	0.0	0.0
OTH MALE GEN	0.0	0.0	0.0	0.0	0.0
KIDNEY	0.0	0.0	0.0	13.4	0.0
BLADDER	0.0	0.0	0.0	0.0	0.0
OTH URINARY	0.0	0.0	0.0	0.0	0.0
MELANOMA SKIN	0.0	0.0	0.0	0.0	0.0
OTHER SKIN	0.0	0.0	0.0	0.0	0.0
BRAIN	0.0	0.0	0.0	0.0	4.8
THYROID	0.0	0.0	0.0	0.0	0.0
BONE	0.0	0.0	0.0	0.0	0.0
LYMPH & RETIC	0.0	0.0	0.0	0.0	0.0
HODG LYMPH	0.0	0.0	0.0	0.0	0.0
LEUKEMIAS	0.0	0.0	0.0	0.0	0.0
OTH LYM & HEM	0.0	0.0	0.0	11.6	16.1
OTHER CANCER	0.0	0.0	0.0	0.0	11.3
OTH BRAIN CA	0.0	0.0	7.2	0.0	0.0
ALCOHOLISM	0.0	0.0	0.0	13.4	0.0
DIABETES	0.0	32.1	0.0	0.0	0.0

(CONTINUED)

AVG ANNUAL AGE-ADJ (1970 US STANDARD) MORTALITY RATES/100,000
NEW MEXICO RESIDENTS, 1958-82, BY ETHNICITY, SEX, AND CAUSE

ETHNIC OTH NW
AND SEX MALE

	YEAR_01				
	1958-62	1963-67	1968-72	1973-77	1978-82
	AGE_RATE	AGE_RATE	AGE_RATE	AGE_RATE	AGE_RATE
	SUM	SUM	SUM	SUM	SUM
SITE					
CIRCULATORY	239.0	134.0	171.5	166.3	128.7
RHEUM FEVER	0.0	0.0	0.0	0.0	0.0
CHRON RHM HRT	0.0	0.0	0.0	0.0	0.0
ISCHEMIC H D	109.0	51.9	45.6	63.5	106.4
HYPERTEN H D	18.5	0.0	27.6	0.0	16.1
HYPERTENSION	0.0	0.0	0.0	0.0	6.1
CEREBROVASC	66.1	66.5	52.2	51.8	0.0
OTH HRT & CIR	45.2	15.5	45.9	50.8	0.0
RESPIRATORY	26.6	17.7	63.7	29.7	21.1
ASTHMA	0.0	0.0	0.0	0.0	0.0
INFLUENZA	21.7	0.0	0.0	0.0	0.0
PNEUMONIA	0.0	17.7	49.4	15.2	0.0
CHR BRONCHI	0.0	0.0	0.0	0.0	0.0
EMPHYSEMA	0.0	0.0	14.2	14.4	0.0
COPD	0.0	0.0	0.0	0.0	16.1
OTH RESP DIS	4.9	0.0	0.0	0.0	4.9
PEPTIC ULCER	0.0	13.7	0.0	0.0	0.0
LIVER CIRRHO	0.0	29.9	0.0	0.0	0.0
NEPHRI -O	0.0	0.0	0.0	0.0	0.0
KIDNEY INFECT	0.0	0.0	0.0	0.0	0.0

(CONTINUED)

MORTALITY RATES

AVG ANNUAL AGE-ADJ (1970 US STANDARD) MORTALITY RATES/100,000
NEW MEXICO RESIDENTS, 1958-82, BY ETHNICITY, SEX, AND CAUSE

ETHNIC OTH NW
AND SEX MALE

	YEAR_01				
	1958-62	1963-67	1968-72	1973-77	1978-82
	AGE_RATE	AGE_RATE	AGE_RATE	AGE_RATE	AGE_RATE
	SUM	SUM	SUM	SUM	SUM
SITE					
PREGNANCY CMP	0.0	0.0	0.0	0.0	0.0
CONGENITAL AN	9.8	0.0	0.0	0.0	3.9
DIS INFANCY	4.9	8.2	19.0	10.7	0.0
SYMP, ILL-DEF	49.3	15.5	0.0	0.0	22.0
OTH DIS, NEC	22.6	6.4	16.4	0.0	45.4
TL EXTERNAL	6.2	23.6	5.3	49.1	37.2
MOTOR VEH ACC	6.2	19.0	0.0	19.7	11.7
OTHER ACC	0.0	0.0	5.3	22.5	0.0
SUICIDE	0.0	0.0	0.0	6.8	21.0
HOMICIDE	0.0	4.5	0.0	0.0	4.4
LEGAL INTRVNT	0.0	0.0	0.0	0.0	0.0

APPENDIX

AVG ANNUAL AGE-ADJ (1970 US STANDARD) MORTALITY RATES/100,000
NEW MEXICO RESIDENTS, 1958-82, BY ETHNICITY, SEX, AND CAUSE

ETHNIC OTH NW
AND SEX FEMALE

	YEAR_01				
	1958-62	1963-67	1968-72	1973-77	1978-82
	AGE_RATE	AGE_RATE	AGE_RATE	AGE_RATE	AGE_RATE
	SUM	SUM	SUM	SUM	SUM
SITE					
ALL SITES	49.1	75.9	136.7	145.0	236.0
INF & PARA DIS	0.0	0.0	5.8	4.3	11.4
TUBERCULOSIS	0.0	0.0	5.8	0.0	0.0
INF & PARASIT	0.0	0.0	0.0	4.3	11.4
TOTAL CANCER	6.2	2.8	10.7	24.1	55.8
BUC CAV & PHAR	0.0	0.0	0.0	0.0	7.8
ESOPHAGUS	0.0	0.0	0.0	0.0	0.0
STOMACH	0.0	0.0	0.0	0.0	0.0
COLON	0.0	0.0	0.0	20.3	0.0
RECTUM	0.0	0.0	0.0	0.0	0.0
LIVER & BIL	0.0	0.0	0.0	0.0	16.1
PANCREAS	0.0	0.0	0.0	0.0	0.0
LARYNX	0.0	0.0	0.0	0.0	0.0
TR, BR, & LUNG	0.0	0.0	0.0	0.0	0.0
OTHER RESPIR	0.0	0.0	0.0	0.0	0.0
BREAST	6.2	0.0	0.0	0.0	4.1
CERVIX	0.0	2.8	0.0	3.8	0.0
CORPUS UTERI	0.0	0.0	0.0	0.0	0.0
OTHER UTERUS	0.0	0.0	0.0	0.0	0.0
OVARY	0.0	0.0	7.9	0.0	0.0

(CONTINUED)

MORTALITY RATES

AVG ANNUAL AGE-ADJ (1970 US STANDARD) MORTALITY RATES/100,000
NEW MEXICO RESIDENTS, 1958-82, BY ETHNICITY, SEX, AND CAUSE

ETHNIC OTH NW
AND SEX FEMALE

	YEAR_01				
	1958-62	1963-67	1968-72	1973-77	1978-82
	AGE_RATE	AGE_RATE	AGE_RATE	AGE_RATE	AGE_RATE
	SUM	SUM	SUM	SUM	SUM
SITE					
OTH FEM GEN	0.0	0.0	0.0	0.0	0.0
PROSTATE	0.0	0.0	0.0	0.0	0.0
TESTIS	0.0	0.0	0.0	0.0	0.0
OTH MALE GEN	0.0	0.0	0.0	0.0	0.0
KIDNEY	0.0	0.0	0.0	0.0	0.0
BLADDER	0.0	0.0	0.0	0.0	0.0
OTH URINARY	0.0	0.0	0.0	0.0	0.0
MELANOMA SKIN	0.0	0.0	0.0	0.0	0.0
OTHER SKIN	0.0	0.0	0.0	0.0	0.0
BRAIN	0.0	0.0	0.0	0.0	0.0
THYROID	0.0	0.0	0.0	0.0	0.0
BONE	0.0	0.0	0.0	0.0	0.0
LYMPH & RETIC	0.0	0.0	0.0	0.0	0.0
HODG LYMPH	0.0	0.0	0.0	0.0	11.4
LEUKEMIAS	0.0	0.0	0.0	0.0	0.0
OTH LYM & HEM	0.0	0.0	0.0	0.0	0.0
OTHER CANCER	0.0	0.0	2.8	0.0	16.1
OTH BRAIN CA	0.0	0.0	0.0	0.0	0.0
ALCOHOLISM	0.0	0.0	0.0	0.0	0.0
DIABETES	0.0	0.0	0.0	15.3	0.0

(CONTINUED)

AVG ANNUAL AGE-ADJ (1970 US STANDARD) MORTALITY RATES/100,000
NEW MEXICO RESIDENTS, 1958-82, BY ETHNICITY, SEX, AND CAUSE

ETHNIC OTH NW
AND SEX FEMALE

	YEAR_01				
	1958-62	1963-67	1968-72	1973-77	1978-82
	AGE_RATE	AGE_RATE	AGE_RATE	AGE_RATE	AGE_RATE
	SUM	SUM	SUM	SUM	SUM
SITE					
CIRCULATORY	6.5	31.1	61.6	60.4	107.8
RHEUM FEVER	0.0	0.0	0.0	0.0	0.0
CHRON RHM HRT	0.0	0.0	0.0	2.9	0.0
ISCHEMIC H D	0.0	31.1	28.6	26.9	71.5
HYPERTEN H D	0.0	0.0	0.0	0.0	0.0
HYPERTENSION	0.0	0.0	0.0	0.0	0.0
CEREBROVASC	6.5	0.0	32.9	30.5	20.0
OTH HRT & CIR	0.0	0.0	0.0	0.0	16.1
RESPIRATORY	0.0	0.0	0.0	8.6	32.3
ASTHMA	0.0	0.0	0.0	0.0	0.0
INFLUENZA	0.0	0.0	0.0	0.0	0.0
PNEUMONIA	0.0	0.0	0.0	8.6	16.1
CHR BRONCHI	0.0	0.0	0.0	0.0	0.0
EMPHYSEMA	0.0	0.0	0.0	0.0	0.0
COPD	0.0	0.0	0.0	0.0	16.1
OTH RESP DIS	0.0	0.0	0.0	0.0	0.0
PEPTIC ULCER	0.0	0.0	0.0	0.0	0.0
LIVER CIRRHO	0.0	0.0	0.0	0.0	0.0
NEPHRI -O	0.0	13.4	16.4	0.0	0.0
KIDNEY INFECT	0.0	0.0	0.0	0.0	0.0

(CONTINUED)

MORTALITY RATES

AVG ANNUAL AGE-ADJ (1970 US STANDARD) MORTALITY RATES/100,000
NEW MEXICO RESIDENTS, 1958-82, BY ETHNICITY, SEX, AND CAUSE

ETHNIC OTH NW
AND SEX FEMALE

	YEAR_01				
	1958-62	1963-67	1968-72	1973-77	1978-82
	AGE_RATE	AGE_RATE	AGE_RATE	AGE_RATE	AGE_RATE
	SUM	SUM	SUM	SUM	SUM
SITE					
PREGNANCY CMP	0.0	0.0	2.8	0.0	0.0
CONGENITAL AN	0.0	5.0	4.8	8.6	0.0
DIS INFANCY	12.3	20.0	4.8	0.0	0.0
SYMP, ILL-DEF	6.5	0.0	0.0	0.0	16.1
OTH DIS, NEC	0.0	3.4	16.4	10.9	0.0
TL EXTERNAL	17.5	0.0	13.0	12.4	12.3
MOTOR VEH ACC	11.0	0.0	5.1	9.0	0.0
OTHER ACC	0.0	0.0	7.9	0.0	4.0
SUICIDE	6.5	0.0	0.0	3.3	4.1
HOMICIDE	0.0	0.0	0.0	0.0	4.1
LEGAL INTRVNT	0.0	0.0	0.0	0.0	0.0

Index

access to health care, 14, 21, 23, 41, 50, 54–60, 65, 76, 78, 151–52
accidents, 113, 119, 124–27
acculturation, 41
age adjustments, 5, 7, 8
age-period-cohort graphs. *See* birth cohort graphs
age-specific trends, and rates for alcohol-related deaths, 109, 110, all-cause mortality, 13, 14, 21, 22, brain cancer, 36, 45, breast cancer, 33, 34, 43, colo-rectal cancer, 31, diabetes, 52, 57, 59, 60, homicide, 135–36, 139, infectious diseases, 66, 70, 71, 72, 74, 75, injuries, 118, 119, 124–28, ischemic heart disease, 84–87, 92, lung disease, 99, 100, 102, ovarian cancer, 45, prostate cancer, 42, respiratory diseases, 99, 100, 102, stomach cancer, 27, suicide, 134–35, 138–39, symptoms/signs/ill-defined conditions, 146–48
airplane crashes, 119
Albuquerque, 4, 90, 91, 104
alcohol consumption, and accidents, 127, 128, all-cause mortality, 21, cancer, 41, 42, intentional injury, 127, ischemic heart disease, 91, 92, motor vehicle fatalities, 126, tolerance to alcohol, 112, tuberculosis, 70
American Indians, and mortality rates for alcohol-related deaths, 108–12, all-cause mortality, 13, 14, 21, bladder cancer, 33, brain cancer, 36, 45, breast cancer, 33, 34, 43,

cervical cancer, 34, 44, colo-rectal cancer, 31, 41, diabetes, 51–52, 54, 59–60, homicide, 135–36, 139, 140, 141, infectious diseases, 65, 66, 69, 70, 71–73, 73–75, 78, injuries, 119, 120–21, 124–28, ischemic heart disease, 83, 85, 91–92, 93, leukemia, 37, lymphoma, 37, 46, ovarian cancer, 36, 45, pancreatic cancer, 31, 32, 41, 42, prostate cancer, 32, 42, respiratory diseases, 98, 99, 100, 101, 104, suicide, 134–35, 137–38, 141, symptoms/signs/ill-defined conditions, 147, 148, 149, 150, 153, 154, uterine cancer, 35; assignment of ethnicity for, 1; diabetes prevalence and, 50; population of, xv; surnames for, 2, 6
Anglos, 111. *See also* non-Hispanic whites
Apache Indians, 72, 75, 93, 127, 137
Arizona, 59, 60, 72, 111, 137, 139
arteriosclerotic heart disease, 84
Asians, 23, 39
asymptomatic prostate cancer, 42
autopsies, 111, 145, 152, 154

Behavioral Risk Factor Survey, 90
Berlin, J. D., 138
Bernalillo County, 73
Bexar County (Texas), 87
birth cohort graphs, 8, for alcohol-related deaths, 109, 111–16, all-cause mortality, 13, diabetes, 52, 53–56, infectious diseases, 66, 69–76, ischemic heart disease, 85, 86–

228 INDEX

birth cohort graphs (*continued*) 91, respiratory diseases, 99–100, 101–4, symptoms/signs/ill-defined conditions, 148, 149–54

birthplace, 2, 4; parents' birthplace, 2, 4

blacks, American population of, xv, and mortality rates for alcohol-related death, 108, brain cancer, 36, breast cancer, 34, cervical cancer, 34, 44, diabetes, 50, homicide, 135, 141, infectious diseases, 71, leukemia, 37, lymphoma, 37, prostate cancer, 42, stomach cancer, 27, 39, symptoms/signs/ill-defined conditions, 146, 148, 151, uterine cancer, 35; general cancer incidence, 23

bladder cancer, 33, 43

brain cancer, 36, 45

breast cancer, 33, 34, 43; birth cohort graphs for, 39, 40

Britain (British study), 57

broad ligament cancer, 35

bronchial cancer, 99

bronchitis (chronic), 99

burn-associated deaths, 119

California, 87, 98, 108

cancer, 23–47; potentially curable, 23; screening for, 34

cardiomyopathy, alcoholic, 113

cardiovascular disease, 59, 87, 91, 93

case-control study for ethnicity, 1

case-fatality ratios, for cancer, 23, diabetes, 50, 57, infectious disease, 72, 74, 78, suicide/homicide, 140

cause of death, and alcohol, 108–16, 128, all-cause mortality, 12–22, cancer, 23–47, diabetes, 50–61, infectious diseases, 65–79, injuries, 118–29, ischemic heart disease, 83–94, malignant neoplasms, 24, respiratory diseases, 98–105, suicide/homicide, 132–41, symptoms/signs/ill-defined conditions, 145–58; categories and codes for, 1, 9, 14, and alcohol, 108, 113–16, 128, cancer, 24, diabetes, 50, 54, 61, infectious disease, 66, 78, injury, 118, 119, ischemic heart disease, 83–84, 93, respiratory disease, 99, 101, symptoms/signs/ill-defined conditions, 145, 151; death by legal intervention or execution, 133; medical history and death, 145; underreported deaths, 34, 114, 140; unknown or uncertain death, 14, 145. *See also* death certificate data

cervical cancer, as curable, 23

cervix uteri (cancer), 34, 43–44

chlamydia trachomatis, 69

cholesterol, 89, 92

chronic disease, 21, 41

chronic obstructive pulmonary disease, 21

cigarette consumption (smoking), 21, 41–44, 57–59, 90, 92, 98, 100–104

cirrhosis of the liver, 108, 111–12, 113, 114

classification of diseases (cancer), 38. *See also* cause of death, categories and codes

clinical characteristics (diabetes), 57

cohort effect, 103

Colombia, 39

Colorado, 40, 57, 98, 102

colo-rectal cancers, 27, 31, 41; birth cohort graphs for, 35, 36, 37, 38

comparability ratios for cause of death codes, 9, 66, 84, 133

Cook County, 112

coronary artery disease, 83, 84

coroners, county, 154

corpus and other uterus cancers, 35, 44

cultural factors (beliefs), 54, 58, 60, 75, 138

curanderos/curanderas, 58, 76, 153

death certificate data (coding), 1, 38, 46, 50, 60–61, 93, 101, 114, 145,

154, 157. *See also* cause of death, categories and codes
death rates and age-specific rates, 8
death with no signs of disease, 145
declining/decreasing mortality rates for all-cause mortality, 13, 14, 21, cervix, uteri, 34, 44, colo-rectal cancers, 41, diabetes, 52, infectious diseases, 65, 66, ischemic heart disease, 83, 85, 86, 88–89, 91, lymphoma, 37, motor vehicle fatalities, 126, respiratory diseases, 99, 103, stomach cancer, 27, 38, 40, symptoms/signs/ill-defined conditions, 147, uterine cancer, 35
delay in treatment, 23, 76
Denver, Colorado, 40, 102
diabetes, 50–61; cancer mortality and, 41, 42; complications of, 59; ischemic heart disease and, 90, 92; prevalence rates for, 50, 53, 59; severity of, 57; tuberculosis and, 70
diagnosis, and brain cancer, 45, cervical cancer, 44, colo-rectal cancers, 41, diabetes, 55, 57, leukemia, 46, pancreas cancer, 41, prostate cancer, 42, respiratory disease, 101; cancer incidence ratios and, 38; changes in diagnoses, 8
diarrheal disease, 66
diet (nutrition), and cancers, 39, 41, 42, 43, 44, infectious diseases, 65, ischemic heart disease, 91, 92
drowning, 119, 125, 127
dysplasia, 44

echinococcus granulosis, 69
economics: the cost of injuries, 118. *See also* socioeconomic status
education, health, 104
emphysema, 99
encapsulated organisms, 73, 75
endometrium, 44
enteric infections, 69
environment and injury mortality, 127
epidemiology of cancer, 47

Eskimos, 72, 139
estrogens, 44, 45
ethnicity, 1, 115
etiologic agents, for cancer, 38, 41, 42, 44, 45; for meningitis, 71
excessive cold, exposure or neglect, 120, 121, 125, 127
eye examinations, 58

fallopian tube cancers, 35
falls and injury mortality, 119, 125, 127
female breast cancer, 33, 34, 39, 40, 43
fertility, 43, 45
fibro-cystic disease, 43
firearms, 127, 139, 140
fire-associated deaths, 119
folk healers, 76, 153; medicine men, 60, 75, 153; traditional healers, 58, 60, 153

gastritis, alcoholic, 113
gender-specific trends, and mortality rates for alcohol-related deaths, 109, 110, all-cause mortality, 13, 14, 21, bladder cancer, 33, 43, brain cancer, 36, 45, colo-rectal cancer, 31, diabetes, 51, 59, homicide, 135–36, 139, 140, infectious diseases, 66, injuries, 119, 121, 124, 125, 127, ischemic heart disease, 84–85, 87, 88, 90, leukemia, 37, pancreatic cancer, 31–32, 41, respiratory disease, 98, 99–100, 102, 103, stomach cancer, 27, 39, 40, suicide, 124, 134–35, 137, 138–39, symptoms/signs/ill-defined conditions, 147, 148, 149, 157; ethnicity and, 5, 6; intercensal populations and, 7
genetic factors, and cancers, 41, 42, 43, 46, diabetes, 57, infectious diseases, 73, 75, leukemia, 46
geographic factors, 2, 55, 57, 60, 78, 128, 152–53

hanging, as a means of suicide, 138
healers, folk and traditional, 58, 60, 76, 153; medicine men, 60, 75, 153
health beliefs, 54, 58, 60; cultural factors (beliefs), 75, 138
health care, 12, 21, 38, 54, 55, 58, 60, 145. See also access to health care
health problems. See alcohol consumption; cigarette consumption (smoking); geographic factors; injuries; poverty; socioeconomic status
health service, lack of coverage for, 55, 76, 151–52
health status, 14, 127, 145, 152
heart disease, 83–84; all-cause mortality and, 21. See also ischemic heart disease
hematopoietic disease, 46
hemophilus influenzae, 69
hepatic alcohol dehydrogenase activity, and alcohol tolerance, 112
herpesvirus infections, 69
high-risk groups, for cancers, 32, 39, 40, 41, 42, 44, alcohol consumption, 110, drowning, 127, homicide, 135, suicide, 138. See also risk factors
Hispanics, and mortality rates for alcohol-related deaths, 108, 109, 110, 111–12, all-cause mortality, 13, 14, 21, 22, bladder cancer, 33, brain cancer, 36, 45, breast cancer, 33, 43, cervical cancer, 34, 44, colo-rectal cancers, 31, 41, diabetes, 51–54, 57–59, homicide, 135–36, 139–40, 141, infectious diseases, 66, 69, 70–71, 73, 73–76, injuries, 119, 124, 125, 127, ischemic heart disease, 84–86, 87–90, leukemia, 37, lymphoma, 37, ovarian cancer, 35–36, 45, pancreatic cancer, 31, 32, prostate cancer, 32, 42, respiratory diseases, 98, 99–100, 101, 102, 103, stomach cancer, 27, 39–40, suicide, 134–35, 138, 141, symptoms/signs/ill-defined conditions, 147, 148, 151–52, 153, 157, uterine cancer, 35, 44; assignment of ethnicity for, 1; cancer incidence for, 23; diabetes prevalence and, 50, 57; populations of, xv, 2–6

Hodgkin's lymphoma, 36, 37, 45
homicide, 113, 119, 124, 127, 132, 135, 139, 140
Hopi Indians, 59, 111
hormonal factors, 42
human papillomavirus, 44
hypertension, 90, 92

immunization, 21, 65
incarceration, as a risk factor for suicide, 138
incidence rates, for cancers, 23, 38, of the breast, 43, cervix, 44, colo-rectal, 41, lung, 98, prostate, 42, stomach, 39–40; for leukemia, 46; for suicide, 140
increasing mortality rates for alcohol-related deaths, 110, 111, all-cause mortality, 14, bladder cancer, 33, brain cancer, 36, 45, breast cancer, 33, 43, cervix uteri, 34, colo-rectal cancer, 31, diabetes, 51–53, 57, 60, homicide, 135–36, 139, 140, injuries, 125, ischemic heart disease, 85, 92, leukemia, 37, 46, pancreas cancer, 31, 41, prostate cancer, 32, 42, respiratory disease, 99, 102, 103, stomach cancer, 40, suicide, 134, 135, 138, symptoms/signs/ill-defined conditions, 147, 149, 157
Indian Health Service (IHS), 21, 60, 69, 72, 74, 78, 91, 110, 139
infant mortality, 13, 21
influenza, 66, 73
injuries: alcohol and, 113; all-cause mortality and, 21; intentional injury, 121, 124, 126; suicide as injury death, 140
insurance, lack of, 55, 76, 151–52
intermarriage, 2

International Classification of Disease (ICD), and cause of death codes, 1, 9, 14, 24, 66, 78, 83, 108, 119, 132, 145, 146, 157; and changes in disease codes, 66, 78
ischemic heart disease, 22, 54, 59, 83–94, 147, 148, 149, 157

kidney infection, 66

language barriers, 2, 4, 58, 60
leukemia, 37, 46
life expectancy. *See* years of potential life lost
lifestyle, 65, 70, 75
lipoprotein, 89, 92
liver biopsy, and alcohol tolerance, 112
liver disease, 108, 111, 114
lung cancer, 21, 23, 98–103
lung diseases, 98, 99
lymphoma, 36, 37, 45

maiden names, effect on census data, 2, 4
malignant neoplasms, 24
medical history, 145
Medicare, 59
medicine men, 60, 75, 153; folk and traditional healers, 58, 60, 76, 153
medicines and drugs, 127
meningitis, 66, 69, 71–73
microvascular diseases, 59
morbidity from ischemia, 92
motor vehicle fatalities, 113, 118, 119, 124–25, 125; suicide as, 140
myocardial infarction, 92

National Cancer Institute (NCI), and Surveillance, Epidemiology, and End Results Program (SEER), 6
National Center for Health Statistics, and vital statistics report, 9, 139
National Institute on Alcohol Abuse and Alcoholism, 128

natural causes of death, 145, 157
Navajo Indians, 59, 60, 71–72, 74, 75, 78, 92, 111, 152
nervous system cancers, 36
Nevada, 128
New Mexico Bureau of Vital Statistics, 83
New Mexico Health and Environment Department, 1
New Mexico in Maps (Williams), xvi
New Mexico Tumor Registry, 23, 43, 46, 47
non-Hispanic whites, and mortality rates for alcohol-related deaths, 109, 110, 112, all-cause mortality, 13, 14, 21, 22, bladder cancer, 33, 43, brain cancer, 36, breast cancer, 33, 43, cervical cancer, 34, colorectal cancer, 31, diabetes, 51–54, 55, 57–60, homicide, 135–36, 139, 140, infectious diseases, 66, 69, 70, 73, 74–75, injuries, 119, 124, 125, 126, 127, ischemic heart disease, 84–87, 87–90, 93, leukemia, 37, lymphoma, 37, ovarian cancer, 35, 45, pancreatic cancer, 31–32, prostate cancer, 32, 42, respiratory diseases, 98, 99–100, 101, 102, stomach cancer, 27, suicide, 134–35, 137, 138–39, symptoms/signs/ill-defined conditions, 147, 148, 150, 157, uterine cancer, 35, 44; assignment of ethnicity for, 1; cancer incidence in, 23; populations of, xv
Northwest Coast Indians, 137

obesity, 43, 44, 90, 92; attitude toward weight, 58, 60
objective ethnic identifiers, 2, 6
occupational exposures, 42, 43
Office of the Medical Investigator (OMI), 127, 139, 140, 154, 157
osteoporosis, 127
Otitis media, 69
ovarian cancer, 35, 45

pancreas cancer, 31–32, 41–42
Papago Indians, 60
Papanicolaou smear technique (Pap smear), 43, 44
parasitic diseases, 66
parents' birthplace, 2, 4
pedestrian fatalities, 113
period effects, and mortality trend data, 8
Pima Indians, 59
plague, 69
Plains Indians, 60
plasma cholesterol, 92
pneumonia, 66, 69, 73
polyneuropathy, alcoholic, 113
population density, 57
population estimates, xv, 2–8; intercensal estimates, 7
poverty, 21, 41, 138. *See also* socioeconomic status
predictive index for death, 57
prevention, 21, 141
prostate cancer, 32, 42
psychosis, alcohol, 113
Pueblo Indians, 75, 93
Puerto Rico, 39, 112
pulmonary, chronic obstructive disease, 98, 99, 100, 101, 102

questionnaire for ethnicity, 4–6

racial classification, 6
radiation, 43, 45, 46
rectum and colon cancers, 27, 31, 41; birth cohort graphs for, 35–38
regional trauma systems, 128
rehabilitation, and alcohol use, 21
renal disease, 59
residence location as a factor, 12, 21. *See also* geographic factors
risk factors, for breast cancer, 43, cervical cancer, 44, children 153, diabetes, 59, fall-related mortality, 127, influenza, 78, injury, 128, ischemic heart disease, 89–93, leukemia, 46, pancreatic cancer, 41, tuberculosis, 70, uterine cancer, 44
road conditions, 126
rubber workers and prostate cancer, 42
rural areas, 54, 60, 76, 126, 140, 147, 148, 151, 152–53

San Antonio Heart Study, 57, 58, 59
San Diego County, 58
sanitation, 65
San Luis Valley, 57
screening for cancer, 34
seat belts, nonuse of, 126
serum cholesterol, 89
serum triglycerides, 89
sex-specific trends. *See* gender-specific trends
sexually transmitted diseases, 44
sexual practices and cancer, 42, 44
Sioux Indians, 139
social attitudes, and alcoholism, 112
socioeconomic status, 40, 43, 44, 54, 60, 89, 126, 138, 151; poverty, 21, 41, 138
Spanish origins, 2, 4–6
stomach cancer, 27, 38–41; birth cohort graphs for, 31–34
stress, as a cardiovascular disease risk factor, 91, 92
subjective measures of ethnicity, 2, 6
suicide, 132, 134–35, 140; alcohol and, 113; injury and, 119, 124, 126, 127
surnames, 1, 2, 4–6
Surveillance, Epidemiology, and End Results Program (SEER), 6
symptoms, signs, and ill-defined conditions, 93, 101, 115

Tecumseh, Michigan, 59
Texas, 40, 50, 57, 58, 87–90, 98, 108, 111, 151
total external mortality, 119
trachea cancer, 99

trachoma, 69
trauma care, implementation of regional systems of, 128
treatment: effect of improvement in treatment, 8, 41, 42; effect upon cancer mortality rates, 23; of infectious diseases and decrease in infant mortality, 21; with traditional medicines, 58, 60, 75
tuberculosis, 65, 66, 69, 70–71
Tucson Indian Health Service Area, 139

unattended deaths, effect upon death certificate coding, 154
uncertain or unknown deaths, effect upon death certificate coding, 14, 145
underreported deaths, 34, 114, 140
unintentional injury, 124–26, 127
United States Census Bureau, 2–8
United States whites, and mortality rates for alcohol-related deaths, 108, all-cause mortality, 21, brain cancer, 36, 45, breast cancer, 33, cervix uteri, 34, 44, colo-rectal cancer, 41, diabetes, 50, 51, 52, 53, homicide, 135, 140, infectious diseases, 65, 71, 73, 74, injuries, 119, 124, 125, ischemic heart disease, 85, 87, 92, 93, leukemia, 37, lymphoma, 37, ovarian cancer, 35, prostate cancer, 32, 42, respiratory diseases, 98, 99, 102, stomach cancer, 27, 39, 40, suicide, 134, 139, symptoms/signs/ill-defined conditions, 146, 147, 148, 150, uterine cancer, 35; age adjustments for, 8; cancer incidence for, 23; diabetes prevalence for, 50, 59
urban areas, 147, 148, 153
uterus, cancers of, 34, 35, 44

vaccination, 78
violent death, 132; intentional injury, 121, 124, 126
viral infections, 46
vital record certification, 41, 45

weight, attitudes toward, 58, 60; obesity, 43, 44, 90, 92

years of potential life lost (YPLL), 21, 50, 126, 136

Zuni Indians, 75, 137

Contributors

Thomas M. Becker, M.D., Ph.D., associate professor of medicine and adjunct assistant professor of anthropology, University of New Mexico Medical Center and the Department of Anthropology, and New Mexico Tumor Registry. He is the recipient of the American Cancer Society Junior Faculty Research Fellowship.

Janette S. Carter, M.D., assistant professor of medicine, University of New Mexico Medical Center, and director, General Medical Clinics and Diabetes Clinic, Veterans Affairs Medical Center, Albuquerque, New Mexico.

Liza D. Chavez, M.P.H., M.D., internal medicine resident, Santa Clara Valley Medical Center, Santa Clara, California.

Rita S. Elliott, M.A., technical editor, Department of Epidemiology, New Mexico Tumor Registry.

David K. Espey, M.D., staff physician, Department of Internal Medicine, Gallup Indian Medical Center, Gallup, New Mexico.

Charles R. Key, M.D., Ph.D., professor of pathology, University of New Mexico Medical Center, Department of Pathology, and medical director, New Mexico Tumor Registry.

Corinne Peek, B.A., doctoral candidate, University of California at Los Angeles, School of Public Health, Los Angeles, California.

Jonathan M. Samet, M.D., M.S., professor of medicine, and chief, Pulmonary and Critical Care Division, University of New Mexico Medical Center.

C. Mack Sewell, Dr.P.H., M.S., state epidemiologist of the State of New Mexico, Santa Fe, New Mexico.

Charles L. Wiggins, M.S.P.H., doctoral candidate, University of Washington School of Public Health.